SO-AUH-880

# 52
## DAYS

## The Cancer Journal
### A True Story

## Jordan Lane

iUniverse, Inc.
Bloomington

**52 Days: The Cancer Journal**
**A True Story**

iUniverse books may be ordered through booksellers or by contacting:

iUniverse
1663 Liberty Drive
Bloomington, IN 47403
www.iuniverse.com
1-800-Authors (1-800-288-4677)

ISBN: 978-1-4759-6277-2 (sc)
ISBN: 978-1-4759-6279-6 (hc)
ISBN: 978-1-4759-6278-9 (e)

Library of Congress Control Number: 2012921990

Printed in the United States of America

iUniverse rev. date: 11/15/2012

# Contents

# Foreword

*Doctor Shane Dormady, MD, PhD*
*Summer 2012, Mountain View, California*

There are only a handful of exceedingly rare diseases whose diagnoses can engender as much fear and anxiety as the diagnosis of cancer. The word "malignancy" alone is so pervasively menacing as to conjure the image of a malevolent being crawling through a loved one's body…or the darkest of poisons seeping through their veins.

However, after practicing oncology for a very short period of time, it becomes clear that some cosmic or spiritual scale does exist to help even the odds when we are at our weakest. There is a light that lives and breathes, casting out the darkness and dispelling the shadows. A light so powerful that it can shine with curative brilliance.

As an oncologist begins their career, they are certain that this light is a random and unpredictable entity, largely dependent on the scalpels, electron beams and chemotherapy used by themselves and other colleagues as they battle cancer.

After some time, the maturing oncologist realizes that all of the radiation, chemo and surgery in the world cannot explain the miracles bestowed upon certain patients. But this evolving practitioner still struggles to determine why the light of cure remains such a fickle ally.

More time passes, and the oncologist realizes that the light is not sparked by evolving therapeutics...not sparked by unraveling the genetic code that creates the human machine. No, the light is something that goes beyond...transcends calculations and chemicals...transcends the human *machine* and unlocks the human *spirit*.

My own career as an oncologist is firmly rooted in Western ideologies, deductive reasoning and basic science. In college, I majored in classical mythology and biology. In medical school, I studied for years to achieve an M.D. and Ph.D. I am now board certified in internal medicine, hematology and medical oncology. I did not do any electives in spiritual healing, alchemy or voodoo.

But even with such sound, comprehensive training in medicine and the biomedical sciences, my first decade as a practitioner of clinical medicine has been humbling. Humbling because I now know that there is only one explanation for watching a patient with stage IV lung cancer receive the most standard of treatments...yet go into complete remission for years and decades. One explanation for the patient whose liver is riddled with metastatic pancreatic cancer but needs just 12 weeks of therapy to cause the disease to evaporate and subsequently travel the world disease free for 4 years (and counting).

One explanation for how a woman with leukemia can suffer a life-threatening clinical collapse, spend 52 days in a teaching hospital and then be found enjoying her grandchild's basketball game 7 years later, completely cured.

This singular explanation is really a recipe of sorts and the four ingredients consist of trust, love, hope and will.

Trust...that your doctors will go to any length to ensure that you get the best, most compassionate and technologically advanced care that modern medicine has to offer. Trust that when they look at you, they see a member of their extended family and that they will be there for you day or night.

Love...the love of one's family which is sometimes the only wind that can blow into the sails of an otherwise defeated patient, allowing the patient to fight on knowing that no matter what turn is taken, there will be two, three or even fifty pairs of hands pulling you out of the fire and onward to better days.

Hope...arguably the most powerful ingredient. All of the treatment in the world will fail without hope. I see this time and time again. If there is one patient reading this anywhere, please promise to never lose hope. Miracles do happen! Stay on your current treatment long enough to be eligible for a new experimental medication. Recycle chemotherapy that worked previously to make it to your child's wedding. Believe that there is always a way to defeat cancer.

And finally, will. To all of my patients, I thank you for allowing me to be part of your life. Thank you for allowing me to do my best to help you, to heal you and, yes, to love you. Thank you for showing me what true courage is as you face your own mortality on a daily basis and tirelessly fight on. Thank you for showing me what it means to have the sheer *will to live*...standing in the face of your disease and saying, "Cancer, do your best...I'm not going anywhere today!"

To patients everywhere, I swear that I believe in more than the science and textbooks. The light does exist and it takes every ounce of trust, love, hope and will we have to keep it shining.

Never stop, always believe. Miracles do happen.

# Preface

*Jordan Lane*
*June 18ᵗʰ 2005, Stanford Hospital, Stanford, California*

I was slouched in a chair in the surgery waiting area of Stanford Hospital reflecting on what we just witnessed and the horrible agony that my wife's family was experiencing. I also contemplated the pain and strife that was sure to come. I knew that our lives were forever changed and I had no idea what the future held or why we got to where we were, but I did know that cancer was culpable and this killer is ruthless. I was also keenly aware that the next seconds, minutes, hours, days, weeks, months and years would be pivotal to our family's future and important to document. This time in our lives, no matter how difficult or what the outcome, needed to be remembered. I retrieved a scrap of paper and an old Bic from the front pocket of my black Timberland backpack and began to document the experience of my mother-in-law's battle with cancer. The result of this endeavor is *52 Days: The Cancer Journal*. My purpose in writing this is to educate, inform, and instill hope in those whose lives have been rocked by cancer. Each day we are steps closer to death than the day prior. Some days we are closer to death than others.

***Cancer By The Numbers*** (http://www.cancer.org)

- Men 1 in 2 and Women 1 in 3 - Lifetime Probability of developing Cancer
- 1,638,910 - Estimated US Cancer Cases in 2012
- 66% - Cancer Survival rates for White Americans
- 58% - Cancer Survival rates for African Americans
- 577,190 - Estimated US Cancer Deaths in 2012
- 1,500 - Estimated US Cancer Deaths per day in 2012
- 173,200 - Estimated US Cancer Deaths from tobacco use in 2012
- 33% - Percent of US Cancer Deaths in 2012 from obesity, physical inactivity and poor nutrition
- 29% - Percent of men who have cancer who will die from lung & bronchus related cancer
- 14% - Percent of women who have cancer who will die from breast cancer
- $226.8 Billion - The National Institute of Health estimate of the over-all costs of cancer in 2007.

## What Is Cancer?

Cancer is a group of diseases characterized by uncontrolled growth and spread of abnormal cells. If the spread is not controlled, it can result in death. Cancer is caused by both external factors (tobacco, infectious organisms, chemicals, and radiation) and internal factors (inherited mutations, hormones, immune conditions, and mutations that occur from metabolism). These causal factors may act together or in sequence to initiate or promote the development of cancer. Ten or more years often pass between exposure to external factors and detectable cancer. Cancer is treated with surgery, radiation, chemotherapy, hormone therapy, biological therapy, and targeted therapy.

## Author's Note

*52 Days: The Cancer Journal* is written from my perspective and interpretation of the situation as I experienced it. I attempted to avoid embellishing others' conversations and thoughts that I did not experience directly. I am not a member of the professional medical community and am not affiliated with Stanford Hospital; however, I strived to express the medical situations as accurately as possible based on my understanding of the situation.

# Thursday June 2nd, 2005

*"You gain strength, courage and confidence by every experience in which you really stop to look fear in the face." -Eleanor Roosevelt*

"Ring, ring. Ring, ring." I did not look toward the phone as it rang. I was focused on the television. I was watching a rerun of a gripping episode of *M.A.S.H* titled "Life Time." In this episode there were two wounded soldiers whose life and death directly affected each other even though they never met and were unaware of their connection.

One badly wounded soldier, who arrived at the mobile army surgical hospital by helicopter, had a severely lacerated aorta. He desperately needed a transplant to survive. This soldier needed a new aorta in less than twenty-six minutes from his arrival to the hospital – the clock was ticking. A superimposed timer counted down onscreen as Hawkeye, B.J. and the rest of the 4077th raced to save the life of the GI. Once the time expired, the GI would die. The doctors and television audience knew how much time remained before it was too late. Unfortunately the M.A.S.H. unit did not have an aorta graft that was large enough for the wounded soldier. As the doctors and nurses brainstormed on how they could try to save the first soldier, another wounded soldier arrived in the compound by ambulance.

This eighteen year-old had a severe head wound. He was a perfect donor for the soldier lacking the aorta. The problem was that the soldier with the head wound was not dying fast enough for the transplant. He was brain dead but not physically dead. The medical staff were waiting and preparing for the one soldier's death which, they hoped, would save the other life. The most touching part of this episode was when the Catholic priest, Father Francis Mulcahy, said a prayer asking God to take one boy's life in order to save the other. This is a difficult prayer for anyone to make, and it must be especially taxing for a priest.

Like most M.A.S.H. episodes this episode's conclusion was satisfying if not particularly happy. One soldier's death barely saved the other's life. However, everyone was still in the grip of an immense, misunderstood and unfortunate conflict.

I also did not answer the ringing phone, because the only person calling at this hour of the evening was usually a telemarketer asking if the owner of the house was available or if I made the purchasing decisions in the family. At this time my wife and I did not have Caller ID. We do now. I would rather not speak to telemarketers and, even though I had seen the M.A.S.H. episode at least three times prior, I did not want to miss any of it. It was a classic, co-written by the show's medical consultant Walter Dishell. The phone stopped ringing and no message was left. I convinced myself that it was a telemarketer since they hardly ever leave messages. My focus went back to the television and the phone was quickly forgotten.

A few minutes later the phone rang again. "Ring, ring. Ring, ring." Again I did not answer. This time, however, I became more suspicious because the home phone rarely rang at that hour, and twice in a row was very unusual. Maybe my wife, Sara[1], was trying to reach me or one of Sara's friends was trying to reach her to set up a tennis match. Maybe it was another telemarketer. Maybe a family member was hurt or needed to speak with me. I was not sure. By the time I decided that I should answer the phone, it stopped ringing and no message was left. My attention went back to M.A.S.H. I did however, take the phone from its holder and placed it on the table in front of the couch in the event that it rang again.

A few minutes later my cell phone rang. This got me off the couch quickly. I walked to a table where my phone lay and I opened the phone to see the number. The number was from the 650 area code, but I did not recognize it. My parents and my wife's parents and various other family members live in the area which that area code covers. Since I did not recognize the number, and my family usually calls the home phone, I did not take the call. I convinced myself that it was a wrong number. Once the phone stopped ringing, no message was left.

Then, a few seconds later, my cell phone rang again. The number was the same one from the 650 area code. This time I answered the phone without hesitation. On the other end was my father-in-law, Bill. I could immediately tell that something was terribly wrong. I felt a pang of guilt for not answering the phones earlier.

He asked me if Sara were there. I replied "No." She was teaching a tennis lesson and would return at about quarter past nine. He paused and took in a shallow breath. I knew that he was about to tell me something that was extremely difficult to say and, I assumed, difficult to hear. He told me that his wife, my mother-in-law Miriam,

---

[1] Many names have been changed.

went to a doctor earlier that day, and they discovered an abnormal mass of tissue above her chest.[2] Bill sounded tired and was getting choked up as he spoke.

I needed to say something remotely intelligent in response to this devastating and completely unexpected news. I asked if there was anything I could do to help. I do not remember the exact response. The call ended with me telling Bill that I would have Sara call him right away when she arrived home. I flipped my cell phone closed.

After the call ended, I took a deep breath, said a short prayer for Miriam, and walked to the kitchen. I went to the garden window above the kitchen sink and peered out. The window faced west and the sun was setting. Large and round, it looked like a giant fiery saucer. There were fluffy white clouds dancing around the setting sun, they glowed red and were scattered across the sky. The sun and clouds were hovering above the Pacific Ocean. It was an absolutely gorgeous scene. I uttered another prayer for Miriam and asked God to aid those who would be affected. I went to the freezer and made myself a stiff drink of cheap vodka and ice. I went back to the couch and placed the sweaty drink on the table. Another episode of M.A.S.H. had begun. I had seen that one also. I turned the television off. I knew my life was about to change.

I picked up the phone and dialed Sara's cell. I knew she was teaching a tennis lesson so I left a voice mail. I remember my message distinctly.

"Hi Honey. It's me. Please come home right after your lesson. I have to talk to you."

---

2 The mass of tissue was overlaying Miriam's clavicle above her sternum and was below her skin. It was not visible with the naked eye.

I hung up the phone and took a deep drink of the vodka and ice. The cool liquid, however, did not quench my thirst. My throat was tight and dry as I tried to clear my mind.

I closed my eyes and replayed Bill's call in my mind. I felt numb and helpless and was trying to determine how I would be able to comfort Sara when I relayed the frightening news. I also wondered what this would mean for our lives. I put down the cold drink, took off my glasses and rubbed my eyes.

Miriam epitomized health. She ate the right foods, exercised regularly, played tennis, took long walks and played with her young grandson. She even had a personal fitness trainer. She was nothing but healthy. For all the years I had known her she had been a fit and active person. I kept trying to reassure myself that the mass was not a concern. Someone so fit and wonderful could not have something seriously wrong. I knew this would most likely not be true. I sat and waited listening to the IKEA clock tick, tick, tick the seconds away as the sun sank into the Pacific Ocean signaling the end of another day.

At around eight-thirty the home phone rang again. This time I did not hesitate to answer. "Hello," I said.

It was Bill. He informed me that he and Miriam were going to bed and to have Sara call in the morning. He also told me I would need to help Sara. I was again lost for intelligent words and said something about being there to help. I hung up the phone knowing that Sara would not wait until tomorrow to call her parents. I suspected Bill knew this as well.

At nine fifteen Sara was not home and I had not heard from her after leaving the message an hour earlier. Her tennis lesson was scheduled to end at nine. I again called her cell phone. She answered and said she'd received my message, was talking to her tennis students, and was on her way home. My voice message did not instill the reaction in her that I thought it would. I thought she would have sensed the urgency and fear in my voice and hurried home. I was mistaken.

I pleaded with her to please hurry home. My voice cracked and quivered as I spoke. Listening to myself speak I sounded like a scared little boy. In many respects I was. Sara picked up on this immediately and now knew that something was wrong. I seldom insist on anything, but when I do, Sara knows it is serious and I mean what I am saying. She asked what the matter was and all I could mumble was to please come home. When I hung up the phone I walked to the back door, anticipating her arrival.

When I saw her walk up the steps from the garage toward the back door I opened the sliding glass door and screen door to let her in. She looked at me with shifting, inquisitive eyes. I knew she had a million questions and thoughts swimming in her head. I was acting out of character with the cryptic phone message and abrupt follow-up asking her to come home immediately.

I assisted her with her large tennis bag. This bag held the tricks of her trade – tennis balls, a couple of rackets, a change of clothes, a bag of snacks and water bottles. I frequently joked with her about the weight of her cumbersome tennis bag. It was heavy.

Once the bag was off her shoulders I held her close to me and looked deep into her striking blue eyes. Holding her, I told her that a mass of tissue was found above her mom's chest. Before I could say any more she broke down and began to sob, "No, no, no." All I could do was hold her.

I knew Sara was not expecting me to say that about her mother. I imagined she was relieved to know what the news was, but at the same time she was terrified.

Holding her tight, I tried to comfort her as tears and "no"s continued to flow. I told her about the two phone calls with her dad and how he said he would talk to her tomorrow, and that they did not know any more than that the doctors had found a mass. They did not know what the mass was. The word cancer was not mentioned.

I knew that Sara was going to (and should) call her parents immediately. And that was what she did.

Sara spoke with her dad first and her mom second. I do not recall the entire conversation but it was very serious and exceptionally melancholy. I left the room for most of the call because I wanted to give Sara and her parents' time together on the phone. Miriam was going to Stanford Hospital the next day to be assessed by specialists. She had gone to a local community hospital earlier that day and was not satisfied with the experience. Stanford seemed like the better option.

Once Sara hung up the phone we went to the computer and made plane reservations to fly from Los Angeles to San Jose the next morning. I do not recall if we ate dinner that night.

~~~~~~~~~~~

I would later learn how the mass was discovered and why Miriam was going to Stanford Hospital instead of the closer community hospital. Here is the story I pieced together based on various conversations and from personal observations.

Miriam had a regularly scheduled general physical with a doctor she had been going to for some time. Neither she nor Bill was particularly fond of this doctor, but like many bad habits, it can be difficult to change physicians even if the care provided is not up to par. Miriam thought the doctor was tolerable, but Bill suggested that there could be better options.

Bill sensed that something might not be right with his wife and insisted that he go with her to the appointment. There had been a handful of instances in the past few weeks where Miriam felt short of breath. She was also using multiple pillows at night to prop up her head when she slept. These pillows helped her breathe easier. Being short of breath and using multiple pillows to sleep were not normal for Miriam. However, these symptoms did not seem to suggest that there was anything life threatening occurring in Miriam's body. Maybe she'd caught a cold. Maybe it was nothing at all. I did not know but I am also not a medical professional.

Bill waited in the lobby as Miriam was seen by the doctor. After five minutes, the doctor and Miriam rushed out of the office. The doctor suspected that something was horribly wrong and told them to immediately go to the hospital. It was fortunate that this doctor did sound an alarm and insisted that Miriam visit a hospital. Bill took Miriam across the street from the doctor's office to a local community hospital. After waiting, filling out seemingly endless forms, and talking to various people Miriam was seen by a doctor. The doctor ordered that an X-ray be taken of her chest. The X-ray results showed that there was clearly a mass of tissue, but because of the X-rays' lack of detail, nothing more could be determined about the mass. Miriam, Bill, the doctor and nurses knew that mass was there, but did not know what it was or what to do about it.

During the process of having the X-rays taken and then analyzing them, one of the technicians told her "good luck." This comment was unexpected and upset Bill and Miriam. It sent them into a mental tailspin. *What was she talking about? Miriam was healthy and strong. She only had trouble sleeping. Nothing was wrong, right? Why does she need luck?* They were told to go back to the waiting room, relax and wait. They were getting very nervous, worried and scared.

After a long while in the bustling waiting room, the physician told Miriam to wait and see what happened and come back in a couple weeks. This doctor also gave them a name of another doctor that they could follow-up with. Maybe the mass was nothing. He was not sure. The X-ray was not definitive or conclusive. The recommendation was to wait and see and call the other doctor.

Bill and Miriam were not in favor of this recommendation, especially after the offhanded remark by the technician. They insisted that the doctor perform additional tests to learn more about the mass and if it was harmful, and asked that a CT scan be performed. The doctor agreed but the procedure had to be cleared by the insurance carrier. After contacting the insurance carrier in Omaha, Nebraska by phone, the representative for the carrier refused to cover the test. This upset Bill as he went back and forth with the nurses and the insurance company about getting the test completed. Three hours later the test was performed. Regardless, Bill and Miriam left the community hospital. They had hopes of getting another opinion at Stanford Hospital. They were not going to wait two weeks.

Stanford Hospital is a private hospital and is considered one of the best in the country, if not the world. It is also where Bill and Miriam first met over forty years ago. Miriam was a nurse. The hospital is located on the campus of Stanford University, in Palo Alto, California. In 2012 *U.S. News & World Report* recognized Stanford Hospital and Clinics as one of "America's Best Hospitals." The news magazine evaluated 4,825 U.S. hospitals in 16 medical specialties, such as cardiology and neurosurgery, for its 2011-12 "best hospitals" survey. Only 140 hospitals performed well enough to rank in even one specialty. Stanford Hospital and Clinics was named to the magazine's honor roll, which recognizes hospitals that rank at or near the top in at least six specialties, demonstrating a breadth of excellence. *U.S. News & World Reports* also ranked Stanford number one among all hospitals in the San Jose metropolitan area.

The Stanford Hospital medical staff consisted of 1,910 doctors and over 1,000 interns and residents. There were also 2,000 nurses and 1,000 volunteers at the hospital. Volunteers performed approximately 85,000 hours a service each year. Stanford Hospital admitted over 24,000 patients for in-house care per year. The hospital also saw over 50,000 emergency patients and over 550,000 outpatients each year. However, like any reputable, busy hospital, it could be difficult for patients to make an appointment. Scheduling an appointment at Stanford could take time. Bill and Miriam did not want to experience another hectic day in a hospital waiting room, so Bill made a phone call to a friend, John.

John lost his wife to cancer a few years earlier and was a capacious donor to Stanford University. John's wife was treated at Stanford Hospital. John asked one of the doctors from Stanford, Doctor Fisher, to call Bill that night at 8:00. After speaking for a few minutes, Doctor Fisher arranged for an appointment at Stanford for Miriam at 2:30pm the next day and asked Bill to gather all of the X-rays and other information and bring them to the appointment. Their team of doctors would evaluate her condition.

During the conversation it was clear that Doctor Fisher was an expert. He asked relevant and appropriate questions and knew what Miriam was experiencing. The shortness of breath and using the pillows at night were clear indicators of a serious medical problem. He determined that Miriam needed to be seen at the hospital immediately, the next day.

This five minute phone call with Doctor Fisher from Stanford helped put Bill and Miriam at ease. They finally got to speak to someone who knew what they were experiencing and empathized with them and addressed many of their questions. At the same time this call must have instilled fear and worry in Bill and Miriam, at something so horrific that I cannot possibly express it in words. The doctor insisted that Miriam see him the next day. Getting special treatment at a hospital is comforting, but it also usually means you have a dire situation and you need the most assistance.

# Friday June 3rd

*"The oldest and strongest emotion of mankind is fear, and the oldest and strongest kind of fear is fear of the unknown." -H. P. Lovecraft*

Sara and I woke up early and drove to the Furama Hotel from our home in El Segundo, California, an unpretentious town in the sprawl just south of Los Angeles International Airport (LAX). El Segundo was incorporated on January 18, 1917. The population was 16,033 as of the 2000 census. The most common story of how the city received its name is that in 1911 it became the site of the second Standard Oil refinery (now Chevron) on the West Coast of the United States. LAX borders El Segundo to the north, the beautiful Pacific Ocean is to the west, the 405 Freeway is to the east and the oil refinery is to the south. El Segundo gained some notoriety from the 1990 song by hip-hop group A Tribe Called Quest titled "I Left My Wallet in El Segundo."

The Furama Hotel was located north of LAX and has since been leveled, which is for the best. It was an odd airport hotel, disorganized, and there were always problems with guests and rooms. I once saw a coroner's van carting someone away from the hotel. It was a strange hotel for the coastal region of Los Angeles.

Sara and I usually parked our car at the hotel and took the hotel shuttle to the airport. This way we did not need to deal with parking at LAX, taking a cab, or bothering a friend to take us and pick us up. Also, taking a cab to the airport can be a hassle. Cab drivers leaving LAX are notorious for getting upset with their riders if they only wish to travel to nearby locations like El Segundo. This day was not any different. We parked the car and took the Furama airport shuttle to LAX.

El Segundo is so close to the airport that the southern runway borders the town. We could almost see the pilots' faces from the balcony of our condominium. We would be delighted to walk to and from the airport but unfortunately there was not a safe passageway, and the stigma that Los Angeles public transportation is inefficient is, unfortunately, true.

I have taken cabs from LAX to El Segundo where the driver becomes extremely perturbed to learn that I was only going to El Segundo. Most taxi drivers wanted to go farther so they could collect a higher fare. Currently there is a rule that the minimum fare for a cab leaving LAX is $17.50. I assume this was instituted to placate the angry cab drivers who were asked to drive to a location near the airport. The cabbies felt like they were being cheated.

When we arrived at LAX terminal one, we tipped the hotel shuttle driver a couple dollars, went through the long and winding security line, and waited at the gate for our flight. While we were sitting in the Southwest waiting area at LAX, Sara got an overpriced coffee and a bagel from Starbucks. I was not hungry.

People-watching is a favorite pastime of mine. This activity is especially interesting at airports, which are a great social equalizer, especially in

Los Angeles. The affluent, middle class and poor live in close proximity to one another in Los Angeles but they are separated by freeways, fences and other manmade barriers. This is not the case at LAX. There are not many class barriers in the security line or the waiting area at the gate. I have seen my share of movie stars, celebrities and sports personalities at LAX. This day would not be any different.

In the Southwest Airlines waiting area I recognized that one person waiting for a flight was the actor who played Wayne Arnold on the popular television show, *The Wonder Years*, from the late '80s and early '90s. The actor who played Wayne is named Jason Hervey. Wayne was Kevin's older and usually obnoxious, but amiable, brother. The actor looked similar to the way he did twenty years earlier. He sat in a chair talking on his phone, eating something and waited for his flight just like everyone else. No one paid much attention to him other than a few quick glances, discreet pointing and whispers.

We queued up to board the plane when the Boeing 737 jet arrived at the gate. We were in boarding group A. Standing behind us was an older gentleman from the nearby town of Palos Verdes, a few miles south of El Segundo. He began chatting with Sara and me. He played tennis and knew some of the same people as Sara from the tight-knit Southern California tennis community. He talked about how he was going to San Jose and then to Monterey to check on rental property he and his wife owned. He inquired as to why we were going to San Jose. We looked at each other and responded "family stuff." We boarded the plane bound for San Jose. The chatty gentleman sat three rows ahead of us talking someone else's ears off for the entire flight.

Once we landed, my mom picked us up at the San Jose Airport and dropped us off at Sara's parents' home. Sara's parents and my parents live in Los Altos, about a twenty minute car ride from the San Jose

Airport and a fifteen minute car ride from Stanford Hospital. Los Altos is a city at the southern end of the San Francisco Peninsula, in the San Francisco Bay Area. The population was 28,976 according to the 2010 census. Most of the city was developed between the 1950s and 1970s and was formerly an agricultural town but is currently mostly residential with a quaint downtown and scattered shopping areas. The town is considered one of the premier areas of the Bay Area due to its low crime rate, excellent schools, steadily high housing prices and fantastic weather.

When we arrived, Bill was home and he looked exhausted. He offered us a quick hello as we placed our suitcases in the guestroom. He apologized that he did not know where the sheets or pillows were. Miriam usually took care of organizing the guestroom. We said we would be okay and would figure it out.

Sara and Bill went to the hospital while their Tibetan terrier, Mandy, and I were going to pay a visit to the vet. Mandy had been relentlessly scratching a spot on her back which was now raw and infected.

Mandy and I took one of the Mercedes and headed toward the vet. I had never taken Mandy to the vet before but apparently she loved going and they loved having her. As we approached the office Mandy became extremely anxious and excited. She pushed her wet nose against the car window and wagged her tail vigorously. I took a wrong turn and she let me know it by barking and glaring at me as if to say, "Wrong way, Knucklehead." After a quick U-turn I pulled into the veterinarian office parking lot, hooked Mandy up to the leash, and took her into the office.

Once inside the office the veterinarian examined Mandy. The vet scrutinized the bumps she had been scratching. The bumps were oozing puss and looked awful. After performing a thorough analysis of the dog, the vet told me that these bumps could either be a serious cancer that would demand a lengthy and dangerous surgery, or they could be caused by a minor infection and could be removed in a simple procedure.

The last thing we needed was the dog to have cancer as well.

The vet took a biopsy of the scratched area and asked that someone call her later that day to get the results. I thanked her, was handed a large plastic collar to place around Mandy's neck to prohibit her from scratching, and picked up medication for the infection. Mandy and I drove back to Bill and Miriam's house.

Once we returned home I placed Mandy in the backyard, secured the plastic collar around her neck so she could not scratch the bumps, and made my way to Stanford Hospital. I called Sara and she told me where Miriam's room was. Her room was number forty in the lower level of the hospital in the Cancer Center. It was in this phone conversation that I first heard Sara use the "C" word. The Cancer Center sounded like a horrible place.

Room forty, like many other rooms in the Cancer Center, was specially designed to accommodate patients who needed to keep their contact with outside air, and subsequently outside germs, to a minimum. The air pressure forced out instead of pushing in or being neutral. When the doors to the room were ajar, outside air could not enter the room since the pressure was constantly pushing out. To enter this special room one had to first go through one set of heavy wooden doors. These doors led to a small vestibule with a sink, hand soap, paper supplies, and hand sanitizer. The next set of doors in this small washroom led to the hospital room. It was a rule that one had to sanitize their hands each time they entered or exited this room and they needed to make sure one set of doors was closed before the other was opened. Hand sanitizer would become a creature comfort and mandatory commodity that is still used in the family. I am not convinced of the product's illness-killing or preventative power or overall usefulness, but many members of my wife's family use it constantly.

When I arrived at room forty I walked through the first set of doors, washed my hands and peeked through the small window cut into the second set of doors. Sara, Jessica, Bill and Miriam were in the room. Jessica is Sara's older sister. They noticed me and waved me in. I opened the second set of doors, once the first doors closed, and entered the hospital room.

The room was pleasant considering the circumstances. There was a television mounted on the wall, a private bathroom for the patient to use, a sink, a couple of chairs, and a built-in bench to sit on and to place personal items. Miriam had plenty of magazines and books spread out on the bench and placed around the room. The reading material and the television helped keep her occupied and her mind off the cancer.

After hellos and small talk, I learned that the next day there was going to be a biopsy of the mass of tissue. We were all very nervous about this procedure but tried to keep strong and positive. In the hospital surgeries were called procedures. At first calling everything a procedure felt foreign, but after numerous procedures this word became second nature. Procedure is a much softer term than surgery and almost anything would qualify as a procedure. For example, simple tasks like taking one's temperature was a procedure just as performing a risky and complex operation on one's heart was a procedure. Surgery conjures up negative images while procedure does not.

The details of the biopsy procedure Miriam was scheduled to undergo were the following. She was to be moved to an operating room in another part of the hospital, would go under general anesthesia, and the surgeons would remove a small segment of the mass with a scalpel. Once the slice of the mass was removed, the wound would be cleaned, sutured, and bandaged. The biopsy would be sent for analysis to determine the composition of the mass. This process was crucial in not only identifying the makeup of the mass of tissue, but also in determining what type of treatment, if any, would be appropriate. One of the scariest aspects of this procedure was that Miriam had never been under general anesthesia. She never had any major procedures, never had a blood transfusion, never had any major medical issues. All of this would quickly change.

The doctors were genuinely concerned how Miriam's body would react to the anesthesia. The surgeons who would be performing the biopsy met with Bill and Miriam. They told them that there could be adverse effects, even death, if her body rejected the anesthesia or if she were allergic to it. This reality frightened the family.

Looking back, the situation was not too bad if an adverse effect of anesthesia was the primary concern. We learned quickly that Stanford doctors always told the good, bad, and the ugly before any procedure when the patient or their family asked. Also, most procedures include the possibility of death. We made it clear that the doctors, nurses and staff should not hide or gloss over anything they knew regardless of how gruesome or troubling it may be. I do not know if the doctors shared all their fears and concerns, but we had more than enough fears and concerns to go around. I also assume that the doctors needed to provide as many details as they felt necessary to comply with informed consent laws.

Throughout the day in the hospital room various nurses bustled in and out checking on Miriam. They assured us that everything would be fine. I am sure we all appeared overly worried and scared, and we were. The nurses said that a simple biopsy was nothing to fear. It was a standard procedure. I could tell the family had different feelings. Fear was thick and tangible in the air. In a horrible and real way it felt as if we were awaiting a death sentence to be carried out for a gruesome crime that we knew Miriam did not commit but was found guilty. We would thumb absentmindedly through magazines, stare blankly at the television, and try to maintain a normal conversation that would not create tears in our eyes or a nauseous pit in our stomachs. This was a difficult, tense time. Each second ticked away slowly but audibly on the wall clock. Tick. Tick. Tick.

The fact that we were sitting in a room in the Cancer Center at Stanford Hospital with Miriam felt ludicrous. Two days prior, if someone would have told me I would be there, I would've told them there was a better chance of me doing backflips on the moon or winning *American Idol*. But now that we were there, all of us wanted nothing more than to get out, go home, and forget that any of this had happened. The irony of this situation and our fear and loathing of the Cancer Center was that there would be a time in the very near future that all of us would give our right arm to get Miriam back to the Cancer Center instead of being in the ICU. A simple biopsy would be a welcome procedure over the more complex and life threatening surgeries, I mean procedures, which would come.

The nurses were correct. We were being ridiculous. The biopsy was no big deal and was just the tip of the horrible iceberg that was lurking dangerously in our path. Fortunately or unfortunately, we did not realize this. We were trying to comprehend and process the notion that Miriam was in the Cancer Center and that the next morning doctors were going to make an incision into her skin to remove part of a tumor that was growing inside of her. Looking back it was as if we were on a ship frantic about the harmless waves hitting the bow but neglecting to look up and notice the menacing tsunami closing in on us.

My dad visited us at the hospital that afternoon. He is a physician and professor at Stanford University and would become a phenomenal asset. I remember that my dad, Sara, Bill, Jessica and I sat outside of Miriam's room as a nurse tended to her. The five of us talked. We were sitting on a stripped down hospital bed that had been placed in the hall until it was moved to a room when it was needed. My dad was explaining the biopsy procedure to Jessica clearly and concisely. Jessica's eyes welled up with tears as she listened intently to the procedure description.

Jessica quickly adopted the role of information steward. She knew what was scheduled to happen, what it meant, and who was involved. She learned the medical jargon, tracked down doctors and nurses when needed, and asked many excellent questions. Sara and I, on the other hand, listened more and tried to stay on the peripheral. Jessica definitely took the initiative and became a great liaison of information between the doctors and nurses and would pass the data onto her father, Sara, my father, and me.

During this entire calamity I learned a slew of new words and phrases. I now know what an oncologist is and what it means to be neutropenic. Oncology is the branch of medicine that studies tumors and cancer and seeks to understand their development, diagnosis, treatment and prevention. A medical professional who practices oncology is an oncologist. Neutropenia is a hematological disorder characterized by an abnormally low number of neutrophil granulocytes, a type of white blood cell. Neutrophils usually make up fifty percent to seventy percent of circulating white blood cells and serve as the primary defense against infections by destroying bacteria in the blood. Patients who are neutropenic are more susceptible to bacterial infections and without prompt medical attention or monitoring, the condition may become life-threatening. Neutropenia can be acute or chronic depending on the duration of the illness.

After visiting for a while longer and saying goodbye to my dad, Bill, Sara and I went back to Sara's parents' house. Jessica stayed the night with Miriam in her room. She slept on a chair that converted into a short, uncomfortable bed. Before we left the hospital room I attempted to convert the chair into the bed but could not figure it out despite the seemingly clear instructions stitched to its side. After becoming frustrated and giving up, one of the nurses came into the room and after a few seconds he had converted the chair to a bed and had everything setup. I felt foolish that I could not figure out how to convert a simple chair into bed, but there were more important issues to focus on than my pride.

I do not recall what we did for dinner or what else occurred that evening. I did remember, however, to tell Bill that he should call the vet about the results of Mandy's biopsy. I think he called the next day. We were all worried, not just for Miriam, but for ourselves.

# Saturday June 4th

*"Some days there won't be a song in your heart. Sing anyway." -Emory Austin*

Sara and I joined Bill and Jessica at the hospital in the morning as Miriam was being prepared for the biopsy. None of us slept well that night. When Bill did not sleep at the hospital he stayed at the house and would usually go to bed early and then wake up early as well to head to the hospital, which was about a fifteen minute car ride away. Sara and I stayed in a guestroom in the back of the house while Bill stayed in the house itself. The guestroom, which was essentially a pool room with a couch that converted into a bed, provided more privacy than being in the house and was the place we always stayed when we visited. My parents lived about a mile from Sara's parents. Sara's sister, Jessica, lived about a half mile from Sara's parents with her husband James and young son Sammy. Our families were close both physically and emotionally.

Each morning Bill would usually leave Sara and me a Post-It note listing tasks that needed to be done, what his plans were, what should be picked from the garden, what to do with Mandy, what there was to eat, or asking us to call him. The little Post-It notes became our way of communicating when we were not at the hospital. Sara and

I felt that our job was to do what needed to be done not only at the hospital but at home.

Sara and I arrived at the hospital later that morning and we met in Miriam's room. Bill, Jessica, and Miriam were already there. It was tense. We did not talk much as we waited for the nurses to wheel Miriam into surgery.

After a few arduous minutes the time came as two nurses helped prepare Miriam for the move to the operating area. The nurses had to unhook the various monitoring equipment from Miriam, unlock the wheels to the bed, and wheel her out of the room into the hall. It felt like a death sentence was being carried out. There would not be an eleventh hour pardon.

Miriam being wheeled down the hall is an image that will be forever etched in my mind. I was at the back of the bed next to one of the nurses who was pushing the bed. The other nurse was with Sara and Jessica at the head of the bed. This kind nurse was holding them close telling them that everything would be okay. Sara and Jessica were both crying and the nurse was trying to comfort them. Bill was at Miriam's side as she lay in the bed. He was holding her hand and both of them were attempting to hold back their tears.

As we were turning the corner toward the elevator the nurse comforting Sara and Jessica gave the other nurse a smirk as if to say the biopsy procedure was nothing compared to what was ahead. The nurses in the Cancer Center experience the various stages of cancer on a daily basis. They see firsthand the painful effects of chemotherapy, the pain of treatment, the highs, the lows, the victories and the defeats. They knew what to expect, how patients react, and how family members and loved ones react. The biopsy was only a miniscule and relatively easy step in the journey. The fact that we were already a wreck at this early stage did not bode well for the future. *"These people ain't seen nothing yet,"* is what the nurse's face said to the other nurse though her words and gestures only provided comfort. Luckily, I do not think Sara, Jessica, Bill or Miriam noticed the nurse's expression.

We joined Miriam as she was pushed into an oversized elevator that could easily accommodate the size of the rolling hospital bed. We went to the second floor, exited, and said our tear-filled goodbyes as Miriam was wheeled into surgery. We searched for a place to sit in one of the waiting areas.

Stanford Hospital had a variety of strategically placed waiting areas. Most of them contained overstuffed chairs, couches, wooden chairs, tables, and magazines. The furniture was made so that it could be easily moved and rearranged very much like large blocks for preschoolers.

We sat anxiously in the second floor surgery waiting area for Miriam to emerge from the biopsy. This waiting area was the location where family and friends of people having surgery congregated. It was extremely busy and, unknown to us at this time, would be somewhere that we would be spending a good deal of time in the very near future. We would witness a variety of furniture configurations in this area in the weeks to come.

I did not feel comfortable in the surgery waiting room, and I believe Sara, Bill and Jessica also would have rather been in the Cancer Center in the room with Miriam than waiting there. We sat, waited, prayed, chatted and hoped as people moved around us coming and going like turbulent ocean currents. The surgery area was extremely busy and exponentially more stressful than the Cancer Center.

The waiting area would constantly change as the day progressed and someone would come out of surgery and another person would enter. Many of the surgeries were preplanned so the flow of people could be somewhat regulated and anticipated. The families would come and go in carefully orchestrated waves. We overheard many other families' problems, joys, and conversations. The hospital, and especially the surgery area, was extremely active and fluid.

The usual events for a planned surgery were that the patient and someone accompanying him or her would check in with one of the nurses. Once the surgeon was ready he or she would meet the patient and speak with any loved ones who were there. The surgeon would explain the procedure, talk about how long it would take and address questions or concerns. Once the patient went in for their procedure, someone usually waited for them in the waiting area. There were phones that would connect those waiting with the nurse station in the operating room.

Once a procedure was completed the surgeon would emerge and talk to the congregated loved ones. In almost all cases that I witnessed, the surgeon told the eagerly anticipating family that the procedure went as planned. The surgeon would also report that the patient was recovering in the recovery room, he or she would answer questions, and that would be the extent of the exchange. The personal attention that the surgeons gave the patient and the family was extremely reassuring. This personal touch goes a long way in the healing process. It was an amazing sight to see a person's face glow, turning from desperate concern to total relief, when they learned a surgery was a success. I witnessed this countless times during the time I spent in that waiting area. Unfortunately this success was for others, not Miriam.

As we anxiously waited for news of Miriam's procedure, there were an abundance of tears and tense moments. We cried and worried for her safety. We kept a close eye on the surgery room doors waiting for Miriam's surgeon to appear. Our hearts sank each time the doors opened and her surgeon did not appear. The waiting was unbelievably difficult. The future would bring more waiting, worry, tears and pain. I found myself glancing at my watch every minute and the surgery doors every ten seconds. Time inched slowly forward.

This was an extremely difficult and mentally fatiguing day. Little did we know that more difficult times were on the horizon and a simple biopsy would be nothing compared to what Miriam would have to try to overcome. You know you have come a long way when a spinal tap does not make you squirm, four hours of blood transfusions is the norm, and a PET scan is just another test that needs to be administered.

Eventually, to everyone's relief, the biopsy surgery was a success and Miriam returned to her room at the Cancer Center fully awake and aware. The biopsy results would not be ready for a couple of days. This meant more waiting, more worry and more tense moments.

We also learned that Mandy's biopsy from the vet returned negative for cancer. This was a relief and hopefully a positive omen for the future. The veterinarian was going to perform a simple procedure to remove the infected bumps that the Tibetan terrier had scratched. This procedure was scheduled for the following week. This was welcome news that brought much needed relief, like a cool and refreshing rain breaking up an unbearably sweltering day.

# Sunday June 5th

Miriam came home from the hospital! This was a day of anticipation and waiting for the results of the biopsy which would help determine the next steps in the treatment. Miriam spent most of the day resting on her couch while Sara and I spent the day visiting with her, completing various errands, picking vegetables with Bill in the garden and visiting with my parents and siblings. In addition to my parents, I have three brothers and a sister living in the San Jose Bay Area.

Bill had a large and well maintained vegetable garden. This garden was the place where he could relax and occupy himself. It was his solace and passion. He had grown a bumper crop of tomatoes, zucchini and green beans that needed to be picked and tended to on almost a daily basis. My tasks were to ensure that the garden was watered, the vegetables were picked, and that neighbors, family and friends were given the vegetables so they would not go to waste. During a typical spring and summer there would be frequent barbeques where the bounty would be cooked, eaten, shared and enjoyed. Since this was not a typical spring and would not be a standard summer, I ended up giving away as many vegetables as I could. The garden kept me busy and also helped to occupy some of Bill's time and not only provided delicious food but was a well-needed distraction, a source of stress relief and conversation. The mundane can sometimes preserve our sanity.

# Monday June 6th

*"A physician's physiology has much the same relation to his power of healing as a cleric's divinity has to his power of influencing conduct."*
*-Samuel Butler*

One matter I knew Bill was contemplating was who he should tell about Miriam's illness and how to disseminate the news. My policy was not to say a word until I was told I could.

Miriam was going to go before the congregation at Saint Nicholas Catholic Church in Los Altos at the morning mass for the sacrament of the Anointing of the Sick. This public sacrament was performed by Father Gary.[3] Both my parents and Sara's parents were members of this parish and Sara and I were married in this church. Father Gary had officiated the ceremony. The word that Miriam was ill would be out in the close-knit community after this short healing sacrament.

The sacrament of the Anointing of the Sick was extremely emotional. We were in the front left pew of the church. From right to left were

---

[3] Father Gary, who also officiated my confirmation and wedding, was the inspiration for the book and film *The Rite*. *The Rite* describes Father Gary's journey as a Catholic priest becoming an exorcist. Anthony Hopkins stared in the film. Colin O'Donoghue depicted Father Gary.

Jessica's husband James, their eight month old boy Sammy, Jessica, Bill, Miriam, Sara and me. Sara's parents, who attended mass regularly at Saint Nicholas, usually sat in the last pew at the back of the church. Being in the front was a change for them. My parents also attended the mass.

During the mass Father Gary asked us to come forward to the front of the church in front of the altar and form a semicircle around Miriam facing the congregation. Father first anointed Miriam's forehead with holy oil. We did the same. We placed our finger in the oil and then placed our finger on a part of Miriam, such as her arm or shoulder. It was an extremely emotional ceremony.

Anointing of the Sick is one of the seven Sacraments in the Roman Catholic Church. It is associated not only with bodily healing but with forgiveness of sins. Only a priest can administer this sacrament. He anoints the sick person's forehead with holy oil (usually in the form of a cross), saying; "Through this holy anointing, may the Lord in his love and mercy help you with the grace of the Holy Spirit." He then anoints the hands, saying, "May the Lord who frees you from sin save you and raise you up." He may also, in accordance with local culture and traditions, and the needs of the sick person, anoint other parts of the body without repeating the sacramental formula.

The chief Biblical text concerning Anointing of the Sick is James Chapter Five, verses fourteen to fifteen. It reads, "Are any among you sick? Let him call for the elders of the church, and let them pray over him, anointing him with oil in the name of the Lord; and the prayer of faith will save the sick man, and the Lord will raise him up; and if he has committed sins, he will be forgiven."

After the emotional and public mass, Sara and I said our goodbyes at the church. We were heading to the San Jose Airport and flying back to Los Angeles. My mom drove us to the airport. The car ride was quiet and somber. The flight was eventless and involved prayer, reflection, and small talk. We were fatigued.

Once Sara and I landed and gathered our luggage in Los Angeles we started to walk toward the airport shuttle pickup area to catch the next Furama Hotel shuttle. While waiting, I received a call from a company I'd recently interviewed with for an open position. The young lady on the phone said they'd love to hire me and if I accepted the job I would start July 6th. I was delighted and accepted the job on the spot. This was a positive step and I needed all the good news I could get.

We rode the shuttle to the Furama Hotel, found our car and drove home. When we arrived home Sara went to one of her jobs, at the El Segundo Recreation and Parks Department, to check on her tennis class signups for the upcoming summer tennis session where she was the park tennis instructor. I stayed home attempting to revive my neglected and weed-infested garden and began to research the company I'd just joined. I was not certain what website analytics or email marketing were, but this is what the company did and I was determined to learn more. I was a budding gardener but did not have as green a thumb as Bill or the spacious gardening space he possessed. We tried to stay hopeful. The new job looked promising but my garden did not.

# Tuesday June 7th

*"The most important thing in illness is never to lose heart." -Nikolai Lenin*

The result of the biopsy was available. Miriam was diagnosed with a rare lymphatic cancer called T-cell lymphoma. Lymphoma is a type of cancer that originates in lymphocytes. A lymphocyte is a type of white blood cell in the vertebrate immune system. The lymphocyte undergoes a malignant change and begins to multiply, eventually crowding out healthy cells and creating tumors that

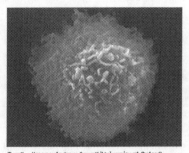

T-cell   (Image: Andrew Sewell/University of Oxford)

enlarge the lymph nodes or other parts of the immune system. There are numerous types of lymphoma. Lymphomas are part of the broad group of diseases called hematological neoplasms. According to The Leukemia and Lymphoma Society about, 71,380 people living in the United States are diagnosed with lymphoma each year. The form of lymphatic cancer Miriam was diagnosed with was extremely rare in adults. When it did occur, it usually occurred in children.

According to the American Cancer Society, "Cancer is a group of diseases characterized by uncontrolled growth and spread of abnormal cells. If the spread is not controlled, it can result in death. Cancer is treated with surgery, radiation, chemotherapy, hormone therapy, and targeted therapy." The overall prognosis for Miriam was not promising. We felt beat, powerless, helpless. Cancer was winning. The death sentence was being carried out.

The treatment for this cancer, like most cancers, was not as simple as taking two pills and calling the doctor in the morning. It was more complex and in line with trying a variety of treatments based on educated guesses, studies and past performance, and using the fine art of trial and error. Doctors might not be sure what doing A would do to the cancer but they try A. If A does not work they try B. Depending on the reactions to A and/or B dictates if C or D is tried. I quickly learned that battling cancer is not a straightforward task. It is like playing a high risk game where one move will dictate the rest of the game and once moves are made, there is no going back or calling "do-over." The doctors at Stanford were fantastic and they worked as a team. Most decisions were not made by one individual but instead by a team of phenomenal professionals. The team did not always agree on the next path to take, but they did respect each other and worked together to provide the best possible care for their patients.

There are many unknowns with cancer and each case and type is unique. This is a primary reason why this disease is so horrible and hard to cure. Cancer is not one disease or condition, but a blanket term for thousands upon thousands of unique conditions that are always mutating and affect people differently.

Luckily the treatment for the stage and type of cancer Miriam was diagnosed with was similar to other types of cancers. The first and second steps in the treatment process were known. After that all bets were off.

The stage of a cancer is a description that expresses the extent to which the cancer has spread. This is usually a number between one and four; with one the cancer is localized to a single part of the body, with two the cancer is localized to a single part of the body but is advanced, with three the cancer is localized to a single part of the body but is advanced and affecting the lymph nodes in a particular way, and with four the cancer has metastasized, or spread to multiple parts of the body. The stage often takes into account the size of a tumor, how deeply it has penetrated, whether it has invaded adjacent organs, how many lymph nodes it has metastasized to, and whether it has spread to distant organs. Staging of cancer is an important predictor of survival, and cancer treatment is primarily determined by staging. Based on what I knew I estimated that Miriam was in stage one or two, unless there was cancer in other parts of her body that had not yet been discovered. I was never told the specific stage Miriam experienced.

Miriam returned to Stanford Hospital where she was assigned to a new room in the Cancer Center, room forty-two, and began to receive treatment. She was admitted to the Cancer Center on a permanent basis for the foreseeable future. Sara and I received frequent phone updates from Bill and Miriam during this exhausting and sad day since we were in El Segundo. Our feelings were exasperated because we were far from Miriam.

# Wednesday June 8th and Thursday June 9th

*"It is normal to give away a little of one's life in order not to lose it all."*
*-Albert Camus*

Sara and I spent the next two days at our home in El Segundo trying to lead as normal a life as possible. Sara kept informed of her mom's progress with frequent phone calls to her parents. I kept in touch with my own parents, exchanging information since my dad visited the hospital frequently and usually had the most recent information.

The facts were usually slightly different depending on whom someone spoke to, but the overall situation was the same. Miriam began treatment for the cancer and everything was moving along as planned. She stayed in the Cancer Center and was constantly surrounded by Jessica, Bill, nurses, doctors and hospital staff. Either Bill or Jessica would sleep in the room at night.

Also, Mandy the dog had her procedure, and it was successful. The veterinarian was able to extirpate all of the infected skin. Once the infection was removed, the skin was cleaned and sutured. Mandy would have to wear a head collar for a few days, but she would heal. This was a much-needed relief for the family.

My garden had become a total loss. I had more weeds than vegetable plants and I could not have cared less. The weeds did not bother me. My mind and heart were elsewhere. Sara and I packed our bags for another jaunt to the Norman Y. Mineta San Jose International Airport.

# Friday June 10th

*"There is nothing permanent except change." -Heraclitus of Ephesus*

At 7:30am Sara and I were driven to LAX by a friend who lived across the street. We went through a long and winding security line, boarded a familiar Southwest Airline jet, and arrived in San Jose. My mom picked us up at the curb and dropped us off at Sara's parents' house where we got one of the cars and drove to the hospital to see Miriam.

Now that Miriam had begun treatment and had a permanent room, our family was becoming a fixture at the hospital. We learned about a fantastic hospitality service offered to patients and their families. A few of these perks include unlimited parking passes, as many Stanford mints as you wanted, and a dedicated individual who worked for the hospital who could be called with questions or concerns. This token of generosity on behalf of the hospital was very much appreciated. Parking fees can add up quickly. In one of the Stanford Hospital parking lots, parking for up to 6 hours costs $6; more than 6 hours and up to 24 hours is $12. More than 24 hours might as well be a second mortgage.

The hospitality program was revolutionary and aimed at not only meeting the needs of the patients but also assisting the family. It was wonderful to have an advocate who could be called when questions or problems arose. We were fortunate to be a part of this program at Stanford Hospital.

We spent the rest of the day at the hospital. Most of this time was in Miriam's room with her. She was awake and in bed except when she had to use the restroom or got her sheets and garments changed. She tried to take short walks periodically but this was rare since she was hooked up to a variety of machines. Some of the machines monitored her vital signs; others gave her fluids, while others allowed her to take medication intravenously. All of the machines fit precisely around a steel pole with wheels. The entire entourage of machines and instruments could roll with the patient as they moved about.

We watched quite a lot of television in the room. This included Miriam's favorite television channel, The Food Network. We read tabloid magazines, and talked about Sammy. I recall thumbing through a *People* magazine that featured the life and death of Pope John Paul II. He had passed away a couple months prior and was on the long and sometimes difficult path to sainthood. Hopefully Miriam would not need saintly intervention, but any help would be appreciated.

My dad came by to say hello and receive an update on Miriam's condition and treatment. Everyone looked forward to his visits. Since he was a doctor and worked at Stanford, it felt like he had divine knowledge or an inside connection that would make everything better. It was interesting to see the looks on the nurses and other doctor's faces when they walked into the room and saw another Stanford physician, with white coat and name badge, in the room. Most of the nurses and doctors looked at him as if to say *"Who are you and what are you doing here?"* But once my dad explained that he was family, everything was fine.

Dad spent about an hour with us. He talked about upgrades the hospital was making to their patient garments, trying to make them more stylish and functional. The new garments would be displayed at a hospital fashion show open to the entire faculty and staff. They were a big deal. Sometimes the little things in life can be quite meaningful and make a significant difference.

After a while Sara and I went back to her parents' house for the night. We ate dinner and went to bed.

# Saturday June 11th

*"Attitude is a little thing that makes a big difference." -Winston Churchill*

Sara and I got up early and completed our habitual morning routine of reading any notes from Bill, scarfing down breakfast, and tending to the garden. The Post-It note this morning simply said, "I am at the hospital." So we joined him there. This was similar to Friday in regards to the activities at the hospital. We talked, visited, said hello to the various doctors, nurses and staff that came and went in Miriam's room, watched television, explored the hospital, and read magazines.

Miriam continued taking the medication she was administered and was checked regularly and consistently by the nurses and doctors. Every fifteen minutes a nurse, doctor or staff member would come into the room, check the various tubes, provide medication, serve food, clean up and ensure Miriam was well. This was the case a minimum of four times per hour, twenty-four hours a day. Quality sleep was impossible with an interruption each fifteen minutes but unfortunately this constant care was essential to fight cancer.

As we were starting to get in a comfortable and familiar routine, the emotions and worries from the biopsy were diminishing. Miriam was following the doctor's orders and the treatment seemed to be progressing positively. The hospital was less frightening.

That evening Sara and I met a friend of mine, John, at a local Mexican restaurant. The restaurant was nearly deserted and we sat at the bar hoping to get a drink before we ate. There were a few other patrons in the bar area but no one was there to wait on us. A waitress walked by but she appeared extremely distraught. After waiting a few more minutes I noticed the same waitress crying behind a divider. She wiped tears from her eyes, took off her apron, and walked out of the restaurant. After that we did not see any other employees. We were uncomfortable and decided to leave. We instead went to a Chili's restaurant. The service was exponentially better. Sara, John and I had a pleasant time catching up. This bizarre evening was a well needed distraction from the hospital and from cancer. We'd confirmed that the world was marching on around us.

# Sunday June 12th

*"Cancer victims who don't accept their fate, who don't learn to live with it, will only destroy what little time they have left." -Ingrid Bergman*

Sunday was very similar to Friday and Saturday. We spent most of the day in the hospital room with Miriam watching television, talking, visiting, and getting her ice cream and ice for her water. We would traverse the hospital, go to the store to pick up sandwiches for lunch, and wander around the Stanford University campus. We were content in the Cancer Center and hospital. The cancer was becoming more remote in our minds as a safe and comfortable routine was established.

The doctors, nurses and other staff were also a part of our routine. We came to know what nurse was on what shift, when the shift ended and what days they were off. Food was delivered every few hours at the same time, and there was always someone coming or going in the room. Everything was on a tight and consistent schedule. A hospital was constantly bustling even in the relatively secluded Cancer Center.

The hospital had many fascinating places to explore. The bottom level had immaculately maintained gardens which included benches and short meandering paths that offered a nice escape from the sounds, smells and pressure of the hospital. Some of the gardens also had small, comforting fountains. All of the floors of the hospital had art hanging on the walls and a variety of sculptures displayed in a variety of locations. Stanford Hospital boasts a collection of more than 500 original pieces of art and 1,600 posters and reproductions. These were displayed in hallways, waiting rooms, hospital rooms and offices. I explored almost every inch of the hospital and saw most of the art. One piece of art that was particularly unique was a bronze sculpture located near one of the entrances. It was of a hat and coat hanging on a wall hanger. Though they were all bronze, they looked remarkably authentic. Quite interesting.

# Monday June 13th

*"Prayer does not change God, but it changes him who prays." -Søren Kierkegaard*

Sara and I took a flight to Los Angeles midday on Monday. We said our goodbyes, got dropped off at the airport and an hour and fifteen minutes later we arrived at LAX planning on taking a taxicab home.

Anticipating a grumpy taxi driver, we waited in line bracing for the worst. When it was our turn to get a cab and the driver asked us where we were going, I reluctantly told him El Segundo. Waiting for a snarky remark like we should take a shuttle, bus or walk, I was surprised when the driver instead responded cheerfully, "I really like Main Street in El Segundo." I smiled as we got into the back seat. The quick ride was relaxing as Sara and I sat in calm silence peering out the window of the cab. This was the most enjoyable taxi ride from the airport I had ever taken. I made sure to tip the driver well.

When we arrived home we unpacked, washed laundry, ate dinner and called our parents. Miriam's condition had not changed. She continued to take the medications prescribed by the doctors, they checked her regularly and consistently, and all seemed to be going well. The shock that Miriam had cancer was wearing off. Outwardly she appeared fine. The doctors and medical team were great and she was in high spirits. Everything was going as well as one could hope considering the situation. This was not to say that we were not worried and fearful, because we were. I had never said so many prayers in my life. So far they were being answered.

# Tuesday June 14th to Thursday June 16th

*"In time of test, family is best."* -Burmese Proverb

The next three days were as ordinary as we could make them. Sara went to work at a local elementary school in the morning where she was a teacher's aide in a classroom with special needs children and taught tennis lessons in the evening. I spent most of this time working around the house. I finished essential housework, paid bills, and tried to enjoy life as much as I could before I started a new job at the beginning of July. I did not bother with my garden, which because of my neglect was now a gnarly patch of weeds.

We were informed that the chemo treatments Miriam received were working and the cancerous mass of tissue had dissipated. It was no longer visible in X-rays! Chemotherapy is not a magic elixir or a mysterious bubbling potion that is ingested to fight cancer. Instead, chemotherapy is a drug treatment that relies on powerful chemicals to kill cells that divide quickly. Chemotherapy is used to treat cancer since cancer cells grow and multiply much more rapidly than most cells in the body. This also means that chemotherapy harms cells that divide rapidly under normal circumstances. This includes cells in the bone marrow, digestive tract and hair follicles. The result of killing these healthy cells includes a decreased production of blood cells, which can compromise the immune system, inflammation of the lining of the digestive track, which can cause nausea, and alopecia/hair loss.

Despite the challenges associated with chemotherapy, the medical team was quite pleased and somewhat astonished with the rapid results in Miriam's cancer. This was very encouraging. The family felt their prayers were answered and all of this would end promptly with Miriam receiving a clean bill of health. However, like many times in life when the best is anticipated, the worst occurs.

# Friday June 17th

*"The greatest mistake in the treatment of diseases is that there are physicians for the body and physicians for the soul, although the two cannot be separated." -Plato*

It was the day of the Spring Sing at the school where Sara worked, marking the unofficial end to the school year. Children, teachers, parents and families attend – it's a community event. This year's theme was Sesame Street Live and featured a variety of songs from the hit PBS television show. My favorite song was "I Love Trash," featuring the crotchety but beloved Oscar the Grouch.

I arrived at the school a few minutes before ten in the morning for the show. It was very cute and well done. I saw people I knew and made plans to play racquetball with Don on Monday evening. Don is the father of one of Sara's tennis friends. After the show I went home and finished packing. Sara and I were flying to San Jose later that afternoon. Sara arrived home around one in the afternoon; we drove to the Furama Hotel, parked our Ford Explorer and took the Furama shuttle to LAX. The routine was followed.

We made our flight and arrived in San Jose. A family friend, Corky, picked us up from the airport and dropped us off at Sara's parents' home. Corky asked if we would like to hang out for a while. We declined and said we would catch up later. We quickly dropped off our bags in the guestroom and hurried to the hospital to visit Miriam.

Sara and I opened the first set of doors to Miriam's room, washed our hands thoroughly in the vestibule, opened the second set of doors and entered the room. We greeted Miriam and took a familiar seat. She looked the same as she did when we last saw her a few days prior. She was pale and weak but in excellent condition considering the circumstances. We told her about our flight, about the Spring Sing and other mundane events. Her dinner had already been delivered and from what I could tell she was not very interested in eating. She picked at the chicken a little, tasted the soup cautiously and carefully pushed the tray away. She was not interested in eating but she did want to take a walk, which was fantastic. The doctors told her that she needed to keep up her strength and stretch her muscles as much as she felt that she was able. The intense drugs not only eradicate the cancer cells, but also healthy cells. Taking a walk would not only be great for her muscles and circulation, but also positive for her mind and personal well-being.

Miriam got herself out of bed, went to the restroom, and prepared for her walk. It was necessary for her to don a facemask when she left the room. This was so she was exposed to a minimal amount of germs in the air as possible. Due to the chemotherapy her immune system was weakening. A common cold could be deadly to someone with an impaired immune system.

I helped Miriam place the large and cumbersome mask over her head. It covered her nose and mouth. She looked like a scuba diver. With the mask concealing her mouth it was difficult to hear her speak and for her to be understood. Sara, Miriam and I slowly exited the room. Miriam did not need to have the IV and other machines attached to her for this walk. We left the machines and monitors in the room. She was free to move without carrying all the equipment and the contraption that looked like a coat hanger with wheels.

We walked cautiously out of the room, took a right out of the Cancer Center, moved down the hallway, past the next wing, past the outside garden and into the main lobby of the hospital. Miriam was extraordinarily weak and had to be extremely careful. The three of us took a short break on one of the soft benches and then continued the journey. We walked all the way to the elevators at the end of the hall. This was the farthest that I had seen Miriam move since she had been admitted to the hospital. As we made our way down the hall we did not speak very many words because it was difficult to understand what was being said through Miriam's mask. She also had difficulty hearing us.

Once we returned to her room and removed the mask she surprised me again. Miriam wanted to sit in a chair instead of going directly to her bed. This was amazing! She not only walked farther than I had seen her walk since she had been in the hospital but now she wanted to sit in a chair. I was astonished at her high spirits and how much she wanted to get well by keeping herself strong. Her attitude was impressive and admirable. She was determined to eradicate the cancer.

Sara and I lingered for a while longer talking and visiting. Bill was coming to the hospital later that night to stay with Miriam. Before we left, Miriam got back in bed and Sara and I made sure she had everything she needed for the night. As Sara and I were exiting the room Miriam looked at us and said, "I love you." This was a very special moment. Little did I know that those three simple but powerful words could possibly have been the last words I would ever hear Miriam speak.

As Sara and I left the hospital we were both in high spirits. Miriam appeared to be doing very well and her spirits seemed to be equally as high as ours. I almost felt happy. Happiness is a feeling that is rarely experienced in the Cancer Center. This was an amazing day.

# Saturday June 18th

*"I have been driven many times to my knees by the overwhelming conviction that I had nowhere else to go." -Abraham Lincoln*

When Sara and I woke up we were still electrified about the great day we had yesterday with Miriam. Sara and Jessica went to the hospital together to have alone time with their mom. I felt a little dejected that Sara did not want me around, but I understood that she wanted to spend time with her mom and sister to celebrate their mother's amazing progress. Instead of going to the hospital I decided to go to my parents' house to see what my brother Matt was doing. Bill, who slept at the hospital that night in the room with Miriam was not at the hospital when Sara and Jessica arrived. He probably went to his massage therapist or ran errands.

When I arrived at my parents' home it was unusually quiet. My younger brother Matt was still in bed and my mom and dad were in Ohio for my dad's high school reunion. Matt had recently graduated from college at Loyola Marymount University (this is the same school Sara, Jessica, Jessica's husband, James, and I graduated from) in Los Angeles and liked to sleep late. He was staying with our parents for the summer and was contemplating enrolling in Law School. I went to the refrigerator to forage for food. I found leftovers, put them in the microwave and sat for a while. I ate my food and thumbed through a recent *Time* magazine. The feature article for the week of June 13th, 2005 was called "Home $weet Home – Why we're going gaga over real estate." The article discussed how home prices were continuing to rise (up a stunning 15% over the past year in June 2005, and 55% over the past five years), where the super-hot markets were, and if homes were an investment to make someone rich. This was during the time when it seemed like everyone was flipping homes, or dreaming about flipping homes, hoping to become wealthy. In hindsight, this was not a positive economic plan.

Around 11 I knocked on Matt's door and asked if he wanted to go to lunch. I was not famished but wanted to get out of the house. He suggested Chinese food. That sounded fine with me. I was in the mood for sweet and sour pork. I went to the bathroom to get ready to go to lunch with Matt. While I was in the bathroom my cell phone rang. It was Sara.

"Hello," I answered.

"Jordan," started Sara. Her voice was hushed and shaky. "Get here now. Something happened." That's all she could get out.

"I'm on my way."

The fact that Sara wanted me at the hospital immediately meant something dreadful had occurred. I told Matt I had to go and I rushed to the hospital in the Mercedes. When I arrived I quickly parked and then speed-walked to the ground level, Wing F, the Cancer Center. As I approached the wing I saw Sara, Jessica, Bill and a hospital chaplain sitting on a bench in the hallway adjacent to the same elevators that Miriam, Sara and I walked past the prior evening.

They were in tears and the chaplain was embracing Jessica. I sat down, was introduced to the chaplain and tried to comfort Sara.

It was explained to me that earlier that morning Miriam had experienced difficulty breathing. Jessica and Sara were with her in the room. They called the nurse a few times. The nurse came each time, checked on Miriam, rearranged the tubes, helped her sit up and left. Sara and Jessica called Bill. The first time they called him they told him he should come soon. Miriam continued to have trouble breathing. Rearranging the tubes and repositioning Miriam did not help. Jessica and Sara knew something was horribly wrong. They called the nurse again and again called Bill. This time they told him to get down there immediately. Miriam was gagging and it looked as if she were choking.

Bill, Sara and Jessica were in the room with Miriam when the Code Blue was called. Code Blue, in my opinion, is the most abominable hospital code. It frequently means that any doctor in the hospital who is available, or the assigned code response team, should get to the called location immediately. A hospital manual states that "Code Blue is often used to represent a real or suspected imminent loss of life – the patient has stopped breathing and their heart has stopped beating." During the time I spent at the hospital I probably heard one Code Blue per day. I also heard one Code Red, which is for fire, and one Code Pink, which is for a missing baby from the nursery or a missing patient. The Code Red was a false alarm and the Code Pink was declared "all clear" by the announcer on the hospital's internal audio system a few minutes after it was announced. I prayed that the child or patient was found safe.

When the Code Blue was called for Miriam it was similar to a frantic scene from the television show *ER*. Fifteen or so doctors and nurses were scrambling into the room trying to revive Miriam. She had labored breathing and then stopped breathing. Sara and Jessica were pushed aside and Bill managed to grab his wife's hand and speak comforting words to her as the doctors tried their best to stabilize Miriam. Sara, Jessica, and Bill were eventually ordered to leave the room.

As Sara, Jessica, Bill and I waited in the quiet hallway all we could do was cry and pray. After a few tense minutes a doctor approached us and shared some information. She informed us that Miriam was being transferred to the surgery wing of the hospital. They had stabilized her enough so that she could be moved. As the doctor spoke, a flurry of doctors and nurses sped past pushing Miriam in her bed. They were wheeling her quickly toward a waiting elevator. I caught a fleeting glimpse of Miriam as the hurried doctors wheeled her away. I surmised the doctor talking to us was there to not only inform us of the situation, but to also prevent us from blocking the fast moving bed and to provide comfort.

I saw that Miriam's eyes were shut and she had a breathing tube down her throat. Fresh blood covered her lips and nose. I surmised that the blood was from the breathing tube being forced down her throat to try to keep her air passage opened to keep her alive, but I was not certain. As Miriam was rushed down the hall I heard the hospital paging system requesting a Doctor Wong. I did not know how this would affect our situation or if this page was related to Miriam, but I said a quick prayer that whoever Doctor Wong was and whomever he or she was going to help, that he or she had God's assistance to do a fantastic job. I pictured Doctor Wong to be an older man with gray hair.

We were notified that Miriam was being taken to the surgery unit by the doctor and that we should move to the surgery room waiting area. This doctor gave a quick, forced smile as she rushed after the gurney carrying Sara and Jessica's mother, Bill's wife and my mother-in-law.

The chaplain strongly suggested that we make our way to the surgery waiting room, which was on the floor above. She suggested this a couple times but none of us responded. We did not want to go to the surgery waiting room. We wanted to go to Miriam's room with Miriam where we could watch TV, talk about the latest celebrity gossip, and feed her ice cream. We were frozen. This was unreal, impossible and wrong. Why did this happen to Miriam? It was not fair, just or right. After more aggressive coaxing from the chaplain we followed her into the now empty elevator up to the surgery waiting area.

The surgery waiting area, which was the same one we waited in during the biopsy, was a place that we would come to know intimately. It would be Camp Miriam for the next few lengthy and taxing days. At first we found the waiting area tolerable. It consisted of a variety of movable, overstuffed and wooden chairs and tables. Since this was a Saturday the area was not exceedingly busy since most weekends were reserved for emergency cases and not preplanned surgeries. We settled toward the end of the room in an area that had stuffed chairs and a foot rest. This was to be our new home.

We did not know what happened to Miriam and the doctors were also unsure. One of the doctors kept us informed with the latest information. However, currently there was no information. I was deducing that possibly she had a heart attack or was choking on food, but I really had no way of knowing. None of us did. Waiting was like a slow and painful torture. I kept replaying Tom Petty song titled "The Waiting" over and over in my head. Here is the chorus:

*The waiting is the hardest part*
*Every day you see one more card*
*You take it on faith, you take it to the heart*
*The waiting is the hardest part*

As we waited, it became apparent that we were not going back to the Cancer Center in the foreseeable future. I offered to collect some items from Miriam's room – her purse, and other personal items. I made this suggestion to not only escape the waiting area, but to allow Jessica, Sara, and Bill time together. The group agreed that it was a good idea to retrieve some of her things, so I went.

As I approached room forty-two in the Cancer Center both sets of doors were wide open and the air conditioner that blew air from inside out was off. This confirmed my assumption that Miriam would not be returning to this room. The room was a disaster. It looked like a powerful earthquake and an F5 tornado hit at the same moment. Everything was thrown to the floor and then moved around chaotically as if it were in a blender. There were various tubes, plastic bags, and other medical supplies open on the floor. I was thankful that Jessica, Bill and Sara did not have to see this mess. It looked like a horribly violent crime scene.

Two maintenance people were cleaning the room. One of them asked me kindly if I were a relative. I replied that I was. The staff member wanted to tell me that I needed to get the items out of there soon so another patient could have the room. But I could tell that he did not want to tell me that. Instead he handed me an empty plastic bag for the personal items. He then placed his hand delicately on my shoulder and gave a wonderfully warm smile. I thanked him with a nod as I scanned the room for what I should bring.

I collected Sara's sunglasses, four or five water bottles, Miriam's purse and backpack, a Stanford Hospital blanket and a stuffed dog from the hospital gift shop which Sara had grown fond of. I left the other items in the room for retrieval at another time. As I was about to exit the room I noticed that a plaster angel that was given to Miriam as a gift for luck was sitting on her food tray. The tray had been shoved aside when the Code Blue was issued. I grasped the angel and analyzed it. This fragile figurine should have smashed to the floor when the tray was shoved to the side, but it was unscathed. This gave me a sliver of hope for the future. If this fragile angel could survive, then so could we. I placed the angel gently on the windowsill near Miriam's other personal items.

~~~~~~~~~~~

As fate would have it, I eventually wound up breaking the angel. It survived the Code Blue but could not survive my clumsy packing. A few days after this I went to retrieve the remaining items that were left in Miriam's room from the nurse's station at the Cancer Center. The nurses were kind enough to pack everything in plastic trash bags and store the bags at the nurses' station. Miriam's room was needed for another patient who was battling cancer.

While I was quickly transferring the various items to a bigger bag, I accidentally dropped a handful of items on to the floor. *Bang!* The items that crashed onto the floor included the angel. The angel's head broke clean off. I felt badly for breaking the angel, but there were more important concerns. I took all of Miriam's items, placed them in the bags, and borrowed a wheelchair from the Cancer Center. I was told in no uncertain terms that this was the last wheel chair that the Cancer Center had and that I had better bring it back immediately. The nurses were reluctant to let me borrow it. After a brief discussion, and my promise to return the chair promptly, I loaded the bulging bags on the chair. I then wheeled everything through the hospital, out the front door, past the smokers,[4] to the parking garage and to one of the cars. I carefully placed the bags in the backseat of the car and started back to the Cancer Center with the empty wheelchair.

On my way to the Cancer Center, as I wheeled the empty chair through the hospitals halls, I noticed a very elderly woman who was having a difficult time walking. She was heading toward a staircase going down and I was sure she would fall. I stopped her and asked if she would like a ride. She stopped, looked at me, looked at the chair and reluctantly agreed with a shrug of her shoulders and a congenial smile. This gentle lady was on her way to visit her husband who was in the Cancer Center. I wheeled her in the chair, showed her where the elevators were and helped her to be reunited with her husband who was battling colon cancer. It was fortunate that I had the empty wheelchair. I did not want to consider what would have happened if that dear old lady tried to climb the staircase down toward the Cancer Center. She would almost certainly have fallen.

After I returned the wheelchair to the anxious nurses, I returned to the car and drove to Bill and Miriam's home. I delicately placed the bags in the garage and quickly went through them, removing anything useful like Miriam's cell phone. I left everything else in the bags in the garage and headed back to the hospital.

---

4 There was a designated smoking area outside the hospital near the entrance we used most often. It was sadly ironic that there would be people smoking so close to not only a hospital but to the Cancer Center.

~~~~~~~~~~~

After selecting a few key items from Miriam's room, I returned to the operating room waiting area. I handed Sara her sunglasses and the stuffed dog which she grasped affectionately. I offered water to Jessica and Bill and they declined with a shake of their heads. Everyone's eyes were bloodshot from crying and our spirits were low. The blanket and waters were laid on the floor as we waited for information on Miriam's condition.

We did not have to wait long. One of the doctors, Doctor Shane, came over and broke the devastating news. The reason Miriam was having difficulty breathing was because her right lung was filling with blood. Internally she was bleeding and was literally drowning from the inside. This explained the progressive choking and the blood around her mouth and nose. He said that the team of doctors was still trying to stabilize Miriam. Once she was acceptably stabilized they would try to stop the bleeding in her lungs if it had not already ceased.

When a person is stabilized this means that they are no longer in imminent danger of death. It becomes relatively safe to perform other necessary procedures. In order to try to stabilize Miriam, the doctors administered drugs that paralyzed her entire body. This ensured that she did not move because motion could proliferate the bleeding and cause other complications.

Later when we asked the doctors how or why the bleeding occurred it was explained that the cancerous tumor had a grasp on various internal organs and blood vessels like an octopus grabbing nearby objects with its strong tentacles. As the tumor shrunk from the chemotherapy and other treatment, it tore the blood vessels, arteries and veins that it surrounded. It is like when a tree is uprooted from the ground. Not only do the roots come out but so do rocks, dirt, pipes and other material entwined with the roots. Doctor Shane explained that once Miriam was more stable an Intervention Radiologist would likely go into her veins to see if he could detect and mend the source of the bleeding. However, this could not be started until she was stabilized. We had to wait until then.

To this point the doctors and nurses have primarily been in the background. I did not know their names, what they were like, or what their specialties were. Jessica kept tabs on most of this information. Now that Miriam had a much more complicated condition from the cancer, I began to know the doctors on a more personal and regular basis. Doctor Shane, for example, was a kind and loving man who had a great bedside manner. He explained things gently, clearly, and professionally. He was a big man with a well-trimmed beard and soft, comforting features. I'm guessing he was thirty to thirty-five years old. His first name was Shane. I do not recall what his last name was. It was always great to see Doctor Shane.

After anticipating, crying, praying and speaking in low whispers to each other, Doctor Shane returned and behind him at a short distance stood a person I guessed to be in his mid-twenties. This man was wearing jeans and a t-shirt and was attentively listing to Doctor Shane as he spoke to us. I could not tell who this other person was and I was not certain if he was with Doctor Shane or merely someone closely eavesdropping on the conversation.

Doctor Shane told us that Miriam was becoming more stable. The drugs to paralyze her were taking effect and he suspected that the bleeding had subsided. He then introduced the jeans and t-shirt man as Doctor Wong.

Doctor Wong stepped a few paces forward. He was pleasant, professional and made me feel more at ease. Apparently this was the same Doctor Wong who was being paged earlier. He spoke with a comforting, balanced tone and explained that the reason he was dressed like he was going out for a casual stroll was because the hospital called him from home on his day off to specifically help Miriam. Doctor Wong explained that he desired to perform a procedure that would hopefully determine the source of the bleeding and halt it. The procedure was called an embolization.

An embolization is a procedure where a substance is inserted into a blood vessel to stop hemorrhaging, or excessive bleeding. Doctor Wong explained that he would insert a tiny camera into a large vein in Miriam's leg and then monitor the camera as it journeyed to the possible source of the bleeding. The purpose was that the doctors could identify the source of the bleeding and then deploy a stent to block the wound and hinder further bleeding.

Doctor Wong gently and courteously explained the side effects of this procedure which included paralysis, death, and other serious complications. If the bleeding source was a major artery and was blocked, there could be other horrible complications such as loss of limbs and organ failure or damage. Also, there might be multiple wounds and it was possible that he could miss some. Bill and Jessica asked numerous questions which Doctor Wong answered. After Doctor Wong explained the risks and answered the questions, Bill signed a liability form. This form stated that Bill would not hold the hospital accountable or liable for the results of the procedure and that he approved the procedure. This was one of many similar liability forms that Bill had to authorize. It was an unfortunate fact that signing forms like these became second nature.

Doctor Wong and his team commenced with the procedure. We waited in silence and prayer.

The procedure lasted a couple of hours and it was successful to a point. Doctor Wong reported that his team did not find the exact location of the bleeding but did block a few minor veins that may have caused a portion of the bleeding. No new bleeding had occurred. It was positive that the bleeding appeared to have stopped on its own. Miriam was no longer drowning in her own blood.

Now that it had been determined that the bleeding had stopped, the main issue was what to do next. Miriam had been heavily sedated as the doctors attempted to stabilize her. She was in a coma. She was stable enough to have the embolization, but not stable enough to return to the Cancer Center and she could not stay in the operating room. It was decided that Miriam was going to be transferred to the Intensive Care Unit.

An Intensive Care Unit (ICU) or Critical Care Unit (CCU) is a specialized facility in a hospital that provides intensive care medicine. These units typically have specialized nurses, doctors and equipment. In the case of the Stanford Hospital ICU, each patient has a full-time, twenty-four hour nurse assigned to them. This one-on-one treatment meant that someone was with the patient at all times. Fortunately for us, the ICU was close to the operating area. We did not need to move from our outpost in the operating room waiting area to be near the ICU.

After more waiting we saw nurses pushing Miriam in her bed from the operating unit of the hospital to the ICU. I got a quick glimpse of her as they wheeled by. She looked horrible. Her eyes were closed, she was pale and motionless. She had more machines hooked up to her than ever before and also had a number of IV's and tubes coming out of her arms and nose. This horrible sight, like other sights from this time, will be with me forever.

Bill went to the ICU to see what he could discover concerning Miriam's condition. He also wanted to ensure he knew what room she was in and introduce himself to the doctors, nurses and ICU staff. It was important to have a good rapport with the hospital staff. Bill made it clear that if anything happened they could and should notify one of us. Someone, be it Bill, Jessica, Sara or me, would almost always be in the waiting room. The primary concern about Miriam's condition was to make sure she was stabilized. She was definitely on the brink of death and her situation was extremely critical. The cancer was no longer the most pressing concern. Keeping her alive was.

After waiting for a while longer at the hospital, I drove alone to Sara's parents' home. Sara, Jessica, Bill and I were planning on staying the night at the hospital in the waiting area and I was going to pick up items for our stay. As I drove to the house I noticed that the street that Bill and Miriam lived on was having a block party. I had totally forgotten about this event that Bill and Miriam helped organize. The neighborhood kids' bikes were decorated and they rode around a large circle following one another and showing off their rides. As I pulled into the driveway Bill and Miriam's neighbor, Jeff, walked up to me.

Jeff was a good friend of the family. He inquired about how things were going with Miriam. At first I was not certain how to respond. I took a deep breath and decided to tell him exactly what had transpired. He was in shock and was speechless for a few seconds. Eventually he said to let him know if we needed anything. I felt like asking him if he happened to have a miracle. He also said that he had something for Miriam. He ran toward his house and disappeared inside.

I walked back toward Bill and Miriam's house. I entered the guestroom and hastily grabbed sweatshirts, toiletries, a pillow, and other items for the night and loaded them into a suitcase. By the time I returned to the car with the suitcase, Jeff was waiting for me. He was holding three large poster boards with all of the neighborhood kids' names on them and other drawings by the children. The posters, in glitter paint and crayons, read: "Get Well Miriam."

Jeff asked me to give Miriam the posters. I took them from him and said that I would. I did not want to tell him that I could not give Miriam these posters then. The ICU had strict rules about bringing outside items into the rooms. Also, Miriam would not be able to view the posters since she was in a deep coma.

I placed the posters in the back of the car with the suitcase. On a future trip back to the house I removed the posters from the car and placed them in the house. I was hoping and praying that one day Miriam would be able to see them. I was not confident that she would.

I slowly waved to the block party as I left the house. I headed to Jessica and James's house to pick up items James had prepared for Jessica. I took these items and returned to the hospital.

When I returned to the hospital I opened the suitcase and showed Sara the items I brought and handed Jessica the items James had packed. Then we waited. Miriam's condition was unchanged. Bill was able to visit Miriam when he pleased despite the ICUs very strict visitor policies. They did not allow large groups in at one time and under no circumstances would anyone be able to stay overnight. Bill said Miriam was still in a medically-induced coma[5] and she was hooked up to a variety of monitors and machines. The nurses and doctors were consistently monitoring her vital signs. She was in horrible condition and could die at any moment.

Coma is a state of prolonged unconsciousness in which the brain is functioning at its lowest level of alertness. Under certain circumstances doctors may induce a temporary coma using a controlled dose of barbiturate drugs. However more likely in Miriam's case they used a drug such as propofol to sedate her. Two common barbiturates used for the purpose of inducing a coma are pentobarbital and thiopental. This type of coma is referred to as a drug-induced coma or medically-induced coma. A medically-induced coma is essentially when the brain is put in hibernation using medication so it can recuperate from trauma, or to immobilize the body. There are numerous risks associated with a medically-induced coma. Pneumonia, for example, can arise because of the patient's immobility. Also, if areas of the brain have been sufficiently damaged due to the severity or duration of the condition which led to the coma, the individual may recover from the coma with permanent disabilities and/or brain damage, or may never regain consciousness.

---

5 It was not clear to me if Miriam was in a medically-induced coma from barbiturate drugs or under procedural sedation from a drug such as propofol. Chemically, propofol is unrelated to barbiturates and has largely replaced sodium thiopental (pentothal) for induction of anesthesia because recovery from propofol is more rapid and "clear" when compared with thiopental. Procedural sedation is probably correct. However, for consistency with what I believed was accurate at the time, I will continue to use the term "medically induced coma" and "coma" knowing that this is probably not accurate and that most likely barbiturates were not used to sedate Miriam.

It's also difficult to determine the severity of a patient's brain damage because traditional neurological tests are not accurate when a patient is heavily sedated. Now that Miriam was stabilizing it was becoming imperative that she awake from the coma as soon as possible. This meant waiting for the medications to wear off or introducing additional medications to help her awake from the coma. There was not a medication that would immediately reverse a coma but some might assist. Studies have found that adult patients who remain in a coma for greater than four weeks have almost no chance of eventually regaining their previous level of function. On the other hand, children and young adults have regained functioning even after two months in a coma. Doctors were anticipating that the drugs would wear off in a matter of hours and days, not weeks. A variety of factors can delay waking up from a medically induced coma including the health, weight, age and other genetic predispositions of the patient. Things do not always go as expected.

My cell phone rang around five-thirty in the evening. My parents were calling from Ohio where they were attending my dad's high school reunion. They called to check on Miriam's condition as they were preparing to go to one of the reunion events that night.

I relayed the horrific story of the day's events. My mom asked why I did not call her earlier. I contemplated calling earlier since I felt that I needed to vent my feelings to someone. I reconsidered because I did not want my torment and pain to burden them, especially since they were far away. I did not want to ruin the good time they were having. Now that I was on the phone with my mom and dad, I told them what had happened and why I had not called earlier. My dad said that he would come to the hospital as soon as he arrived the next day. He thought he may be at the hospital around nine in the evening. They sent their love and I hung up the phone.

I informed Sara, Jessica, and Bill that I'd spoken with my parents and that my father would be at the hospital around nine the next evening. This news saddened them. Nine the next night seemed like an eternity. They wished he was able to get to the hospital before that. It was at this moment that I truly saw the faith and appreciation Bill, Sara and Jessica had for my father. They seemed to have a confident strength when he was present. He brought hope and understanding. These attributes were both extremely helpful to have in our situation.

After hanging up the phone with my parents we thought it would be best if we tried to eat something. Our appetites were almost non-existent. The meal we did share consisted of a hodgepodge of items from a large and beautiful care basket that was delivered to Jessica and James's house from a company Bill used to work for. There was a fruit salad, a risotto dish and rotisserie chicken. No one really ate. We just absentmindedly picked at the food and moved it around on our plates.

As night approached we prepared for sleep. We were going to attempt to sleep in the hospital waiting area. There was not a policy against spending the night and many people slept in corners, on chairs, and on the floor. The hospital was active twenty-four hours a day, year round. This was the status quo. We arranged the chairs, blankets and pillows the best we could. My bed consisted of an overstuffed chair and footrest. I had a pillow from home and a blue blanket the hospital provided. We attempted to rest, but this was futile.

Around midnight a couple of friends of Bill and Miriam's, Sandy and Mike, visited. They lingered for a half hour. It was good to see them. After they left we again tried to sleep.

I do not think I slept that night. The lights were bright and the hospital was noisy, plus the lack of food and abundance of emotions kept me awake. This was an extremely tough day and almost impossible night. I was sure that harder times were to come. And, unfortunately, I was correct.

# Sunday June 19th

*"When you come to the end of your rope, tie a knot and hang on."*
*-Franklin D. Roosevelt*

After sitting restlessly for a few hours, I arose from my chair around 5am. I walked into the bathroom at the hospital, put in my contacts, brushed my teeth, and immediately threw up. My stomach was empty so I had dry heaves. From the lack of sleep, lack of sustenance, and the emotional rollercoaster we were riding, my body needed a release. Once I was done heaving, I brushed my teeth a second time, splashed water on my face, and exited the bathroom.

When I returned to our corner of the waiting area Sara, Jessica, and Bill were awake. Nothing had changed. We packed our things and headed home. The nurses and doctors did not have any updates on Miriam's condition.

Exhausted, Sara and I went to the guestroom at Bill and Miriam's and crawled into bed. I attempted to sleep, but could not. After lying restlessly in bed for half an hour I got up and showered. It was refreshing to be clean. Sara slept for about an hour. She really needed the rest. Once she was awake, we ate and went back to the hospital.

We arrived at the hospital and made our way to the waiting area. We sat in silent thought and reflection for quite a while. Father Gary, our parents' priest who performed the Anointing of the Sick a few days earlier, was going to be visiting later in the afternoon. We were looking forward to his visit.

Bill, Jessica, Sara and I ate lunch around noon. Sara and I picked up sandwiches from a nearby grocery store. We ate in quiet contemplation. Mostly we were exhausted and lost in thought.

Three friends were planning on visiting us at the hospital after lunch. One difficulty we faced was how to treat visitors. Most friends and family naturally wanted to visit and offer their support and comfort. They had good intentions. Many times we did not feel like visiting or talking. Constantly reliving what was happening with Miriam or chattering about other unrelated topics seemed to create more pain and annoyance than comfort. I felt selfish for not wanting to have some people visit while looking forward to others. I did not feel that I should, or could, share my pain and anguish with everyone. I wanted to keep it to myself. Sometimes distance was more comforting than closeness.

I did not feel much like chatting when the three friends arrived. After saying hello and giving them a recap of the situation, the three friends began to talk about things that I did not really care to discuss. They spoke about mundane and distant topics like the weather, movies, traffic, sports.

This visit was exhausting and a little annoying. I did not want to talk anymore but I also did not want to offend anyone by asking our visitors to leave. After a smattering of this idle chitchat Father Gary arrived. The chatting continued until Jessica, Sara, Bill, Father Gary and I excused ourselves and went to Miriam's room.

The ICU staff made an exception and allowed all of us in the room at the same time. I had not seen Miriam since she had been moved to the ICU. She looked horrendous. She was on a ventilator and had numerous machines around her. The machines beeped, and the ventilator moaned as fresh oxygen was pumped into her fragile lungs through the mask covering Miriam's face. She also had a variety of tubes going in and out of her arms. I believe she was close to being on 100% oxygen. This meant that her natural inclinations to breathe on her own were not functioning. The machine was entirely breathing for her. She was in such a deep coma that the sometimes trivial and automatic task of breathing was impossible. If she wasn't in the hospital when her lungs had filled with blood, she would have been dead.

The ICU room was similar to the room in the Cancer Center except that there was a lot more equipment and no place for visitors to congregate or sit. The nurse, who was there for part of the twenty-four hour a day shift, sat in a chair to the left side of Miriam. The nurse faced a panel where he or she could monitor the various machines that were tracking Miriam. It looked like a space station control center.

We packed into the room as Father Gary placed his stole over his neck so that either side draped evenly over his shoulders. He also removed a small canister of holy oil from his pocket. He was going to perform the sacrament Anointing of the Sick on Miriam for the second time.

Once Father Gary had finished the sacrament we all joined hands and said a prayer around Miriam. We hugged each other when we were done. This was a very difficult but necessary ceremony. We needed this for healing and for hope – and maybe we would get a miracle. This sacrament also helped build my personal faith and relationship with God. The time with Father Gary and Miriam allowed all of us a moment to share our grief together. I had learned that the power of prayer was indeed real. We each anointed Miriam with holy oil before leaving the ICU.

After the sacrament was completed, we left Miriam and the ICU. We thanked Father Gary and said goodbyes to our other visitors. Bill walked with Father Gary as he was leaving the hospital. Bill was questioning what was happening to Miriam and why it was happening. Why would God allow something so horrible to occur? Father Gary explained that trying to discover answers for these types of questions was very difficult since many times there were not answers. Father gave Bill special rosary beads with which to pray and meditate. Bill prayed the rosary every day.

Once our visitors were gone we were relieved but fatigued. We went back to our vigil. I also called my friend Don in El Segundo to cancel our racquetball game, which we had scheduled for Monday evening. The Friday earlier and the Spring Sing at Sara's school seemed like a lifetime ago.

Bill and I had a drink of vodka around five-thirty. The daily vodka drink, like the constant use of hand sanitizer and endless amount of water bottles, became one of our creature comforts. Bill enjoyed having a cocktail once a day around five-thirty. This traditionally consisted of a small amount of vodka over ice. That day he had kept himself busy procuring cups and ice. Once five-thirty rolled around he handed me a Styrofoam cup and ice cubes and poured a shot of vodka from a glass bottle of Smirnoff he had in one of his bags. We toasted Miriam and had our little drink.

Also at around five-thirty, a large electronic shade descended, covering the windows in the hospital facing the waiting area. The row of windows was four stories high and went from the ground floor to the third floor. By five in the afternoon the hot sun started creeping through the western facing windows. This heated up the waiting area and nearby hallways and made it uncomfortable and stuffy. The electronic shade provided a needed relief from the powerful afternoon sun. The ritual of the closing shade became very familiar to us over the next few weeks. It broke up the monotony of long days spent waiting and was also something to look forward to.

Jessica's husband, James, made chicken for dinner. He delivered it to the hospital around six that evening. He brought their young son/my nephew Sammy, along with the food. Jessica, James, Bill, Sara and I all ate at the hospital in relative silence. We had a better appetite this night than we did the previous one. It was also good to play with Sammy. He brought relief and a needed distraction. It was comforting to see him smile and he was fun to play with.

Once dinner was complete James and Sammy went home. Bill, Sara, Jessica, and I did more waiting. Every few hours an ICU doctor would find one of us and provide an update on Miriam's condition. Nothing had changed. She was still in a coma and was not showing positive signs of waking up.

My dad came back from Ohio and arrived at the hospital around nine that night. He drove directly from the airport to the hospital. We updated him on the situation. He visited Miriam and introduced himself to the ICU staff, nurses and doctors.

I waited at the hospital until eleven and then went back to Bill and Miriam's to sleep. Sara, Bill, and Jessica, however, slept at the hospital for the second night in a row. I did not feel I could have physically or mentally handled another night in the hospital. I did not know how they could either. This was another difficult day.

# Monday June 20th

*"I have found the paradox, that if you love until it hurts, there can be no more hurt, only more love." -Mother Teresa*

Bill called the house at 6:30am. I had been awake for an hour and answered the phone after the first ring. Bill told me there was no change in Miriam's condition and he had a few errands he wanted me to run. After taking a quick shower and grabbing a bite to eat I was on my way.

The first task, after watering the garden and picking a bushel of green beans, was to deposit a check for Bill. After that I returned to the house and took Mandy to my mom and dad's house. Mandy did not like being left alone all day and my mom was happy to care for her. When I arrived at my mom's house, Mandy was ecstatic to be there and enjoyed the attention that she received. I also learned that my brother Matt had a slight fever and was in bed. I did not say hello to him because I did not want to get any of his germs and then spread them at the hospital. I said goodbye to my mom and Mandy.

My last task was to find a clip that would fit Bill's cell phone so that he could attach his phone to his belt. He had a previous clip but it broke. This seemed simple enough. I had the broken clip and started my quest for a new one. The first stop was the world famous Stanford Shopping Center, which prides itself as the San Francisco Bay Area's premier shopping and dining experience. It has over 140 world class stores including Neiman Marcus, Bloomingdale's and Nordstrom. I, however, did not have any luck finding a replacement phone clip. The store I visited did not have a comparable clip. From there I went to six phone stores without any luck. Apparently this clip was extremely rare. Most of the cell phone stores did not carry a similar clip and did not know where they could procure one. Eventually I went to a drug store and purchased superglue and fixed the clip myself. One of the hinges had broken off. Gluing the clip to the area where the hinge was missing solved the problem.

During my phone clip quest I ran into one of Matt's friends whom he had not seen in a while. His friend was working at one of the many phone stores I visited. I gave the guy Matt's cell phone number. Maybe these two friends could be reacquainted.

I finally made my way back to the hospital. We had sandwiches for lunch. A family friend, Sandy, graciously made and delivered them to us. We ate hungrily for the first time in a few days.

I did not see Miriam on this difficult day. Bill, Jessica, and Sara would see her periodically. This day consisted of a good deal of long faces, prayer and waiting.

Miriam was in stable condition. Her blood pressure was lower than it had been. This was a positive. However, the doctors said that she might have a heart murmur. This was potentially very negative. Murmurs are abnormal heart sounds produced as a result of turbulent blood flow, which was sufficient to produce audible noise. This condition most commonly resulted from narrowing or leaking of valves, or the presence of abnormal passages through which blood flowed in or near the heart. Murmurs were not part of normal cardiac physiology and thus warranted further investigation. They sometimes resulted from harmless flow characteristics of no clinical significance. The murmur could be an indication that the cancer had spread to the heart or it could be harmless. If the cancer had spread to the heart, it would be almost certain that Miriam would die. The doctors simply did not know what the heart murmur meant or if it was significant.

Also, there was an unknown fluid discovered surrounding Miriam's lungs. The doctors were not certain what the fluid was or what, if anything, they should do about it. They were going to take X-rays of her lungs to see if this would help provide them with more information about the mysterious fluid. The worst case would be that her lungs, or a pocket around the lungs, were filling with blood. If this were true then either the old wounds had reopened or new ones had formed. It was also possible that the fluid could be harmless and would drain or clear up on its own. If the fluid did not clear up on its own it would probably need to be removed. Fluid in or around the lungs was generally very bad. If left untreated the fluid could cause the person to drown or could increase the likelihood of pneumonia. The fluid was a frightening unknown that added more complexity to an already stressful and fragile situation.

We began to describe Miriam's illness and the events following it as a complex puzzle. Every day, every hour, every minute would bring a new and sometimes more complicated and unexpected piece to the puzzle. Conditions were constantly changing. If the blood pressure was not a problem, then the heart murmur was a concern. If the murmur was not a problem, then there was an issue with Miriam's breathing. This was a ludicrous time that was always in flux and changing. Any of these puzzle pieces could be deadly.

Later in the afternoon James brought Sammy to the hospital. Sammy was a needed distraction and evoked a plenitude of smiles. He was in a stage of his life where everything and everyone needed a smile and he was used to people smiling back. Because of this he did not fit in very well at the hospital. In the hospital many people did not return his smile. The hospital was generally very melancholy. Regardless, Sammy brought fun and was a welcome distraction to break up the monotonous routine as we sat and waited. During this day we talked, sat, walked and spent time in the chapel.

The chapel was a small room off to the side on the way to the ICU. It contained a row of simple off-white plastic chairs, various religious books and bibles, a small altar and a fountain. The fountain was electric and attached to the wall. It had a small trickle of recycled water coming out of it. This was a peaceful location to relax and be alone with one's thoughts and with God.

While in the waiting area, Bill relayed a few stories about his past experiences in hospitals. He did not like them as a general rule and was squeamish around blood and injury. The story he relayed was about a friend who got hit in the eye with a racquetball. His friend was playing racquetball without protective glasses and got hit square in his right eye. His friend was at the Veteran's Hospital for treatment when Bill visited him. During the visit his friend, who had a patch over his injured eye, removed the patch to show Bill his injury. The injury was the most disgusting, bloody mess Bill had ever witnessed. When Bill saw the grotesque eye he immediately passed out. On the way to the floor he smacked his head on a chair. He earned a slight abrasion on his head. The hospital did not know what to do with Bill since he was not a veteran but was in a veteran's hospital and the hospital was not obligated to treat his wound at taxpayer's expense. After a quick deliberation and a few stitches to Bill's forehead, the hospital staff sent him on his way.

At five-thirty, Bill and I had our daily drink. It was of course enjoyed in a Styrofoam cup over ice. The large shade descended over the hospital windows. These nightly rituals were something to look forward to and brought normalcy and routine to the long, arduous and worrisome days.

My mom made us high roller sandwiches and pasta salad for dinner. I went to her home to pick them up. I then delivered the food to the hospital where Jessica, Bill, Sara, James, and Sammy waited. No one ate very much but the meal was delicious. There was not any news from the team of doctors concerning Miriam's condition. Nothing had improved or regressed since the last update. The medically-induced coma persisted. The reality of death lingered. I waited with everyone until 10pm. After that I went back to Bill and Miriam's to sleep while Sara, Bill and Jessica stayed at the hospital again. They slept on the familiar floor in the bustling waiting area.

# Tuesday June 21st

*"If you're going through hell, keep going." -Winston Churchill*

I woke at 7am, completed a few errands and dropped Mandy off at my mom's house. I arrived at the hospital at 11am where Sara, Bill and Jessica were in the waiting area. There were few significant changes in Miriam's condition this morning but she was more stable than the prior day. Sara, Bill and Jessica said they slept, but not great. I thought they should sleep at home in their own beds to get a better quality and quantity of sleep but I kept this opinion to myself. They were hungry and were going to go to the Bing Dining Room for lunch. I volunteered to guard the seats while they ate. Since this was a weekday and not a weekend, the operating room waiting area was active. Seats in the surgery waiting area were an extremely precious commodity as people waited for loved ones who were in surgery. My task was to try to protect as many seats as I could, which was not always easy. We had one corner staked out and in that corner we had blankets, water bottles, pillows and magazines. I tried to stage the area to make it look like it was lived in and as permanent as possible. This was not too difficult. We were becoming a fixture.

The Bing Dining Room, where Bill, Sara and Jessica were eating and which we recently discovered, was an actual sit down restaurant with waiters, located in the hospital. The Bing had good food and was reasonably priced. It was hidden away on the third floor near the top of the escalators. It mostly served faculty and staff but was open to the public. Most of the patients and their families did not know it existed. In order to find the Bing one had to take the correct escalator to the third floor and open the proper door. Once someone did discover the restaurant they found that it looked like any other casual American restaurant. The Bing offered an escape from the cruel realities of the hospital. The restaurant had indoor and outdoor seating, lovely linens, adequate plates and utensils, and a little carnation in a vase on each table. Since the dining room was located on the top floor, the outside seating area was on the roof and offered a beautiful sky view. The Bing would become a very familiar place for us during the next few weeks. This respite would provide comfort, nourishment, and friendship during the difficult times ahead.

When Sara, Bill and Jessica returned from lunch and reclaimed their seats, I took a walk to search for food. I ended up in the hospital cafeteria. The cafeteria was a standard hospital eatery and extremely busy. Patients, visitors, and staff mingled together in the cafeteria where there was not any preferential seating or anything spectacular about the place. It was your run-of-the-mill hospital cafeteria. There was a wide variety of food. I opted for the special of the day. It was some sort of chicken dish that was covered with peas and light gravy. The special was disgusting but I still managed to eat half of it. I am not sure why I ordered that meal. I did learn that just because it was named special did not make it special. I returned to the waiting area feeling unsatisfied and slightly queasy from my meal.

The rest of the day we waited, walked up and down the halls of the hospital, talked with each other and the doctors when we could and drank water. We always tended to have a cache of water bottles. Water bottles, like hand sanitizer and the daily drink and window shade, were another of our creature comforts and part of our routine. Also, Bill had begun to wander off periodically to take a nap somewhere in the hospital. He could usually find a vacant couch on which to stretch out and take a break. He was always reachable by cell phone if needed.

During the afternoon my dad visited. He asked me if Miriam had spoken yet. The answer was no, she had not, but the question hit me harder than it was intended to. I asked myself – what if she never spoke again? What if she did not get out of the hospital? What if she were on those machines for the rest of her life? What if a doctor walked out to us right then and told us Miriam was dead? I quickly brushed these questions out of my mind and strained to think positively. This question reminded me of the last words that I heard Miriam speak – "I love you."

During the days at the hospital, Bill, Jessica and Sara would periodically visit Miriam in her room. I did not see her unless I was specifically asked. The ICU did not permit a large number of visitors at a time and they also did not permit the visitors to stay in the room for an extended period. They did not want ICU patients to be exposed to outside germs, plus the ICU was not a place for visitors to be loitering. Generally the ICU staff allowed any of us to see Miriam when we desired. But mostly Bill, Jessica, and Sara would visit her. My primary duties were to run errands, care for the garden, make sure Mandy was cared for, protect our camp in the waiting area, and keep friends and neighbors apprised of the situation when needed.

Later this day we finally received news of a change in Miriam's condition. She was still in a coma from the sedation and the X-rays of her lungs showed fluid, but the doctors still could not determine what the fluid was. They decided to wait and see what happened before making a decision about the fluid. On a positive note, we were informed that Miriam was off all of the blood pressure medications. This was great news. I am not clear what type of blood pressure medication she was given and the specific purpose, but the fact that she was no longer administered blood pressure medication meant that the doctors were confident that her body could regulate its blood pressure without assistance. Because of the severity of Miriam's case, any medication that could be discontinued without any adverse effects was positive.

The doctors also informed us that the oxygen level she was given to breathe was lower than before. This was also positive. The lower the oxygen level meant her body had to work more to breathe. The more her body worked, the faster, hypothetically, Miriam would wake up from the coma. Breathing on her own should make her stronger.

Because of this news we were upbeat and optimistic by the end of this day. Every day we tried to take away something that was positive. Examples of positive news we received over the course of the weeks were that Miriam had wiggled her toe, she was taken off the blood pressure medication, or that one of the many scans and tests she had to undergo had come back negative. Negative, in a hospital, was usually positive.

Bill and I had our traditional vodka drink at five-thirty and watched the window shade descend. We left the hospital later that evening. Sara, Bill and Jessica slept at home instead of on the hospital floor. I believe Bill was at a point where he realized that being at the hospital every second might not be positive for his own well-being and Miriam seemed to be in great hands. The nurses, doctors, and staff were fantastic. Bill needed a good night's sleep in his own bed.

# Wednesday June 22nd

*"Once you choose hope, anything's possible."* -Christopher Reeve

We awoke, showered, and prepared for another day. I picked green beans, watered the garden and Sara and I went to a local bagel and coffee shop, the House of Bagels, to get breakfast. We then took Mandy to my parents' and headed to the hospital. We settled into the all-too-familiar waiting area. I did not see Miriam today but Bill, Sara and Jessica did. They said her condition was the same. She was unconscious, hooked up to a variety of machines, and looked horrible.

Later in the morning Sammy and James arrived. Sammy was entertaining and, as always, he was a welcome distraction. At noon we all went to the Bing Dining Room for lunch. We left our camp unguarded in the waiting room and hoped that it would still be there when we returned. The lunch was refreshing. I had the club sandwich with skinny fries. After lunch, at twelve-thirty, I met my dad at the hospital. He drove me to the San Jose Airport. I was going to fly alone to Los Angeles. My mission was to gather more clothing for Sara and myself and to drive back to the Bay Area in our own car. Flying back and forth was getting tedious and expensive.

On the way to the airport my dad and I discussed a variety of topics. We first discussed Miriam. He expressed concern about the unknown fluid that was still surrounding her lungs and about how Miriam was not waking from the sedation. He said that this could be the effects of the drugs not wearing off or it could be a sign that she'd had a stroke or suffered brain damage. These were concerns that would become extremely urgent in the very near future.

He also spoke about how the doctors were giving Miriam solid food through the feeding tube that went from her mouth to her stomach hoping that she would have a bowel movement. This would help keep her intestines and stomach in working order. They had previously been keeping her hydrated intravenously.

Miriam had also been set up with a PICC line. A peripherally inserted central catheter (PICC) line is used when intravenous access is required over a prolonged period of time. This is primarily used for administering medication. A PICC is a long, thin, flexible tube. It's inserted into one of the large veins of the arm near the bend of the elbow, and is then slid in until the tip sits in a large vein just above the heart.

The space in the middle of the tube is called the lumen. Sometimes the tube has two or three lumens. This is known as double or triple lumen. These lumens allow different treatments to be administered simultaneously. At the end of the tube outside the body, each lumen has a special cap to which a drip line or syringe could be attached. There is also a clamp to keep the tube closed when it is not in use.

The primary advantage of a PICC over other types of central lines is that it is easy to insert, poses a relatively low risk of bleeding, is externally unobtrusive, and could be left in place for months to years for patients who required extended treatment. The chief disadvantage is that it must travel through a relatively small peripheral vein and is therefore limited in diameter, and it is also somewhat vulnerable to occlusion or damage from movement or squeezing of the arm. There is also the possibility of infection and blood clots.

Gradually, the conversation with my dad turned from Miriam to my life. My dad told me that I should do what I think was best regarding decisions. He spoke about the time when my mom's mother passed away and how difficult it was on the family. She passed away at an early age from an aneurysm in her brain. An aneurysm is a localized, blood-filled bulge of a blood vessel caused by disease or weakening of the vessel wall. A sad part of my grandmother's unfortunate and untimely death was that the aneurysm that killed her would have been easy to treat today. I do not remember my grandmother, but I wish I could.

The time spent with my father on the way to the airport was very special to me. I am thankful we had that opportunity.

He dropped me off at the San Jose Airport and I was bound for LAX. I hoped that our car was still parked at the Furama hotel and that it had not been towed. I was away longer than anticipated.

As I waited in the San Jose Airport I saw a family eagerly awaiting a loved one where the security checkpoint ended. They had red, white and blue balloons and a sign that read "Welcome Home." This was a little gathering to welcome a soldier home from war. When the soldier deplaned he did not look a day over eighteen. I wondered what his eyes had seen in war and what types of trials and tribulations he'd encountered. I did not receive any answers to my inquiry and I am not sure I really wanted to. I am convinced that war and cancer are similar in many ways. They both should be avoided at all costs, but when one is stuck with them they need to fight like hell to get out and survive.

As I was sitting at the airport I thought about our car, which was hopefully still parked at the Furama. I opened the pocket in front of my Timberland backpack and began to look for the car keys. I could not find them. I searched more. I still could not find them. I started to hatch a ridiculous plan in my head about how I could retrieve the car if I did not find the keys. This involved calling tow trucks, Ford dealerships, plus other tasks I did not have the time or energy to complete.

I called Sara to see if she had the car keys. She did not. I then checked the back pocket of my bag. Low and behold, the keys were there. I was so mentally fatigued that I was not thinking straight. I had placed the keys in the back pocket so I would not forget where I had put them. Then I had forgotten. I tried to relax the best I could before the flight. It was not easy.

Once I landed at LAX, I caught the Furama Hotel airport shuttle and found that the Explorer was right where I had left it. I turned the ignition and drove home. Once there I washed laundry and packed a few clothes for the trip back to Los Altos and Stanford Hospital.

I grabbed two oversized suitcases and decided to pack Sara's clothing first. I was not sure what exactly to bring, so I opened up her dresser drawers and grabbed half of the contents from each drawer and placed it in the suitcase. I then went to the closet and grabbed a few hanging items for her and also placed these in the suitcase. I am not sure what I packed but I hoped it would suffice. Luckily it did. Once Sara and my bags were packed I put them in our Explorer and headed toward the City of El Segundo Recreation Park.

Once at the park I walked to the tennis courts to see how the Round Robin tennis group was doing. A Round Robin was when people play a game of tennis and switch partners and sometimes switch courts. This was a casual event that occurred once a week at the park. The idea was to be able to play with as many different people as you could. Sara usually ran this.

The group had one court with five people and they were doing a rotation. I said hello and gave a report on Sara's mom. Everyone was supportive. My purpose was to make sure the class was still going and that everyone was having a good time. I next called Jamie, who was Sara's boss and friend at the park. I told him that the Round Robin group was fine, and he did not need to worry about showing up to help direct them. I also gave Jamie an update on Miriam's condition. Jamie is a good family friend. He was Sara and Jessica's tennis coach while they were in college.

After leaving the park I ate and went to bed. My alarm clock was set for 5:30am.

# Thursday June 23rd

*"Hope never abandons you, you abandon it."* —George Weinberg

I woke up at 5:00am, a half-hour before my alarm was scheduled to chime. I showered quickly, ate a banana, packed a few more items and hit the road. I was on California highway 105 at 5:24.

I took the 105 East to 405 North which merged with 5 North. I then took 152 West to 101 North to 85 towards Los Altos. I arrived at Sara's parents' house at 10:30 AM on the dot. Five hours was a new record for me on this 400 mile journey. I averaged eighty-five to ninety miles per hour the entire time. This exceeded the speed limit, but I wanted to get back to the hospital as soon as I could. Luckily, I did not run into the California Highway Patrol.

I drove first to Sara's parents' to drop off the suitcases. When I entered the front yard, there were people in the home cleaning, the pool man was around the pool clearing out the filters, a television installation person was finishing up installing a flat screen television in the workout room while another person was on the roof fiddling with the satellite system. There were workers everywhere. It reminded me of the scene in the 1986 comedy *The Money Pit*, starring Shelley Long and a young Tom Hanks, when there was a group of misfits working on fixing a dilapidated home in a disorganized and slightly comedic fashion.

As I walked with the suitcases, around the house to the guestroom, I said hello to everyone. They did not know who I was but did not question that I was there. I then went to the garage and grabbed a few water bottles to take with me to the hospital. My hands were extremely full.

I walked to the Mercedes which I had been using and I noticed that the car was locked but the windows were partway down. The keys were in the house. I thought that if I reached in the slightly ajar windows and unlocked the door from the inside I could place the water bottles in the car and then go back in the house to get the keys. As I reached my hand in the car and pulled the pin to unlock the door, the car unlocked but the alarm began to scream.

I threw the water bottles in the car and ran toward the house to find they keys. As I was running toward the house I ran past the pool man who was leaving. He glared at me as if I were stealing the car. I quickly explained that I had left the keys inside the house. He walked to his truck with a smile. I found the keys and by the time I returned outside the alarm had stopped screaming and the pool man was gone. I locked the car door and went to the Explorer.

I drove the Explorer to my parents' home to drop off a BMX bicycle to my brother Matt which my mother insisted that he wanted even though he said he did not. Matt had the bike at college when he was in Los Angeles and gave it to me to hold. I went inside the house briefly and saw Mandy. I then placed the bicycle in the garage. Mandy was happy to see me and when I left she tried to follow me out the door. I think the dog wanted to go to her own house. She liked my parents' place, but there is no place like home. I was sure the dog also missed Bill and Miriam.

My mom and I talked briefly. She asked me if I was aware that Miriam was in horrible condition and that she could possibly die. I answered yes. I knew all too well the severity of the situation. Tears welled in both our eyes. It is never easy to discuss or contemplate death, but in this case it was cathartic.

I said goodbye to my mom and drove the Explorer back to Bill and Miriam's, got in the Mercedes and headed to the hospital. When I arrived at the hospital I found Sara, Bill, and Jessica sitting in the ground floor waiting area. They had moved from the surgery waiting area. The ground floor had more comfortable chairs, a different view and was not as chaotic as the surgery waiting area. The mood was somber and extremely tense. I handed them water bottles, and was caught up on the events from yesterday while I was gone.

One mildly amusing story relayed to me happened the night before. This was related to the Smirnoff bottle Bill used for the evening drink. Bill had placed the glass vodka bottle in a paper bag. This was his way of keeping it discreet. My mom and dad were visiting at the hospital and as Bill started to walk them out, he stood up and the glass bottle dropped and shattered on the hospital floor. *Crash!* It had broken through the bottom of the bag. The glass was cleaned up and everything was fine. From that point forward Bill used a metal flask for the vodka instead of a glass bottle. It is unusual to see a broken vodka bottle in a hospital.

On a more serious note, that morning Bill had arrived at the hospital early to see Miriam. When he walked to her room in the Intensive Care Unit both doors were wide open and she was not there. The room was completely empty. There was not a nurse, not a bed, no machines, or anything else except for a wall-mounted television, turned off. Bill began to panic and immediately called my dad, who hurried over and asked the nurses what was going on and where his wife was. It turned out that in the night Miriam was moved from the ICU to one floor lower. There was an emergency and the hospital needed to put a critical patient (who had since been moved) in Miriam's room. The hospital staff neglected to notify Bill about the move. Moving a patient is not uncommon since hospitals are constantly in a state of motion. Sometimes the staff does not have the time or resources to track down the family of the patients when a move must be made.

This incident, however, caused us to keep a closer eye on Miriam. Also, my dad got involved to find out how this happened with the ICU staff. This incident was stressful but amicably resolved. Miriam was found and we were more vigilant regarding her location from that point forward.

Also, Miriam being moved from the ICU told me that either her condition was improving, or it was becoming hopeless and the special ICU services might not be beneficial any longer. The doctors and nurses had to move one patient from the ICU, so maybe they chose Miriam because her case was becoming hopeless, because she was not benefiting or improving in spite of the ICU care. I did not share these assumptions or feelings with anyone. I did not know if they were true, but they felt reasonable.

I then had the opportunity to visit Miriam in her room. She looked a great deal better than she did the last time I saw her, two days prior. Her skin tone was not as pale and clammy as it had been before, it was more pinkish and she looked stronger. But she was by no means well. I could have just been wishing that she was looking better when in fact she was not. There were quite a few concerns.

One concern was that she had been off the sedative drugs and was still in a coma. I had lost track of the actual number of days since the drugs were administered. It was possible that her body was taking an abnormally long time to metabolize the drugs and eventually she would awake. It could also mean that she may have had a stroke or other major problem and might never wake up. If the latter was the case then we would be faced with the difficult decision of when to pull the plug and let Miriam die naturally.

The team of doctors had conflicting opinions on what should or should not be attempted to help Miriam wake. One doctor wanted to administer a certain drug, another wanted to try a different procedure, Doctor Shane suggested that they do nothing. His advice was to wait and see. Possibly all Miriam needed was more time. This was the course of action that was taken. Only time would tell if this would be a positive decision. The coma was an extremely serious problem.

The second concern was that her lungs were still surrounded with fluid. The doctors did not know what the fluid was, or if they should let it be or try to drain it. Third, there was talk that her liver could be damaged and was not functioning properly. Liver malfunction could be related to the excess fluid around the lungs and/or the fact that the sedation drugs were not wearing off. The liver plays a major role in metabolism and has a number of functions in the body, including glycogen storage, plasma protein synthesis, and detoxification. The organ also was the largest gland in the human body and was crucial for survival. Liver failure or liver problems could be extremely serious.

Fourth, her right arm had become abnormally swollen and severely discolored. This was indicative of a blood clot. Blood clots were not as serious as brain damage, fluid around the lungs, or liver problems, but they were still a major concern. A thrombus, or blood clot, is the final product of the blood coagulation step in homeostasis. It is achieved via the aggregation of platelets that form a platelet plug, and the activation of the humeral coagulation system. A thrombus in a large blood vessel will decrease blood flow through that vessel. In a small blood vessel, blood flow may be completely cut-off, resulting in death of tissue supplied by that vessel. If a thrombus dislodges and becomes free-floating, it is an embolus.

Miriam not waking up and having fluid around her lungs were problems that could easily take her life. Also, liver malfunction was a cause for concern and could be indicative of other major complications that had not surfaced. The worst that could happen with a blood clot, if it did not become a free floating embolus and enter the heart or other organ, was that she might lose her limb or its functionality. It was mind-blowing that so many things could go wrong at once and that the loss of a limb was the least worrisome problem. Each issue seemed to compound or cause something else. It felt like everything that could go wrong was going wrong except that miraculously Miriam was still alive. There were many more questions than answers. Miriam was still enduring cancer's effects and fighting for her life.

Up to this point there has been very little mention of her cancer. The cancer, however, caused all of these complications. When the cancer cells were hit with the chemo and other drugs, they reacted so positively that they were destroyed extremely efficiently. The mass above Miriam's chest disappeared almost immediately. But when the mass diminished in size, it took with it surrounding tissue and organs. This was what caused the internal bleeding and other complications. The cancer was still in Miriam. Just because the doctors could not find it did not mean it was gone. The cancer was not the highest risk at this time. I knew we were in trouble when a horrible disease like cancer was not the top concern.

Despite the above concerns, there were a few positives that we hung onto tightly like a castaway grasping a lifejacket in a turbulent and shark infested sea. One was that Miriam's breathing was improving. She was still on the ventilator but the level of oxygen she was receiving from the ventilator was less than a few days earlier. The breathing would fluctuate over the next few days and weeks. Two, she was being administered less medications than previous days. This was excellent news. The less medication she had, the less her body needed to process. Three, the feeding tube was working. She was now getting sustenance to hopefully help her body build itself up to become healthy and strong. Four, she was still off of blood pressure medications. This meant her body was able to naturally regulate blood pressure. This was fantastic.

Miriam was scheduled to undergo a CT scan and an ultrasound later that day or the next. The CT scan would be used to hopefully determine if she had suffered a stroke or any brain damage while under the sedation. This procedure should help explain why she was not waking up or at least eliminate reasons why she was not waking. A CT scan is also called a computerized tomography or CAT scan. It is an X-ray technique that produces images of internal organs that are more detailed than those produced by conventional X-ray exams. Conventional X-ray exams use a stationary X-ray machine to focus beams of radiation on a particular area of the body to produce two-dimensional images. But CT scans use an X-ray generating device that rotates around the body along with a very powerful computer to create cross-sectional images, like slices, of the inside of the body. A conventional X-ray of the abdomen, for example, would show bones as well as subtle outlines of the liver, stomach, intestines, kidney, and spleen. A CT scan, however, reveals these bones and organs as well as the pancreas, adrenal glands, kidneys and blood vessels, and all with a higher degree of precision.

The ultrasound was to be administered on Miriam's arm to see if the doctors could locate a blood clot suspected of causing Miriam's arm to swell. Medical sonography or ultrasonography, is an ultrasound-based diagnostic medical imaging technique used to visualize muscles, tendons, and many internal organs, their size, structure and any pathological lesions with real time tomographic images. Ultrasounds have been used to image the human body for at least fifty years. It is one of the most widely used diagnostic tools in modern medicine. The technology is relatively inexpensive and portable, especially when compared with modalities such as magnetic resonance imaging (MRI) and computed tomography (CT).

Ultrasound is often described as a "safe test" because it does not use ionizing radiation, which imposes hazards, such as cancer production and chromosome breakage. However, ultrasound energy has two potential physiological effects: it enhances inflammatory response and it can heat soft tissue. Ultrasound energy produces a mechanical pressure wave through soft tissue. This pressure wave may cause microscopic bubbles in living tissues and distortion of the cell membrane influencing ion fluxes and intracellular activity. When ultrasound enters the body, it causes molecular friction and heats the tissues slightly. This effect is miniscule as normal tissue perfusion dissipates heat. With high intensity, it could cause small pockets of gas in body fluids or cause tissues to expand and contract/collapse in a phenomenon called cavitation. This is not known to occur at power levels used by modern diagnostic ultrasound units, but the long-term effects of tissue heating and cavitation are not known. There are no known harmful effects associated with the medical use of sonography.

Widespread clinical use of diagnostic ultrasound has not revealed any harmful effects, but the possibility exists that biological effects may be identified in the future. Current information indicates that the benefits to patients far outweigh the risks. The results of these tests on Miriam would not be known until later that afternoon or the next day. We prayed that they would be positive.

While in the waiting area, Bill ran into a friend who used to coach the Stanford Men's Basketball team and later worked in real estate with Bill. Bill refereed college basketball for some time and got to know many of the coaches and personnel. This person was at the hospital for his last radiation treatment for prostate cancer. He, as well as my dad, joined Jessica, Bill, Sara and me for lunch at the Bing Dining Room. As usual, we ate outside under the sun. I ordered a mango quesadilla which was the "special" for that day. The cheese was rubbery and the mango was from a can. This reminded me that I was still in a hospital, and for future meals I would stick with the club sandwich with skinny fries and not deviate from that path. This was the second time I ordered the "special" at the hospital. Both times the food was less than appetizing. I hopefully have learned my lesson – avoid anything deemed "special" pertaining to hospital food.

The lunch was relaxing. My dad enjoyed hearing some Stanford basketball history from the former coach and Bill got to catch up with a longtime friend. As we were finishing our lunch we met the CEO of the hospital, Martha Marsh. She was extremely personable and saw to it that Miriam and our family had everything necessary.

After lunch we went back to the waiting area. Sister Barbara, a nun from Saint Nicholas Church, was coming to visit later that afternoon.

She found us in the waiting area. After we exchanged hellos she asked how Miriam was doing and how her spirits were. Bill explained that Miriam was not doing well. Sister asked if she could see Miriam. Bill and Sister Barbara went in to see Miriam as Sara, Jessica and I waited in the small chapel. Bill and Sister prayed together over Miriam. When they returned to the waiting area Sister looked pale and sad. She was shocked to see what critical condition Miriam was in. I was not sure what she was expecting, but what she saw was exceptionally worse that what she had prepared for. All of us went into the chapel and formed a circle.

Sister anointed us with water from Lourdes, France, and we said a prayer for Miriam. The Sanctuary of Our Lady of Lourdes, or The Domain, as it is commonly known, is a place of mass pilgrimages from Europe and other parts of the world. The spring water from the grotto is believed by the faithful to possess healing properties. An estimated 200 million people have visited the shrine since 1860, and the Roman Catholic Church has officially recognized its ability to create miracle healings. This was powerful water.

The prayer session was touching and tears were welling up in all of our eyes as we prayed for Miriam. After a while we said goodbye to Sister. She said she would be back in a few days with communion and she left. She did return, but Sara and I were already in El Segundo when she visited. We returned to the waiting area.

After a while, Doctor Shane provided the results of the CT scan and ultrasound. We were grateful for his information and the promptness with which the procedures were completed. He said that the CT scan did not indicate any signs of stroke. Miriam's brain looked normal to him. He also reported that he believed a blood clot was causing the arm to swell. The ultrasound identified the area of her arm where the clot resided. Medication would assist with the clot and the doctors would know more later. Also, it did not appear that Miriam had any internal bleeding since the initial incident. He was still not sure why there was fluid around the lungs or what the fluid was. They considered draining the fluid but he was not certain at that time and it was ultimately the ICU staff's decision. Doctor Shane said that he was "hesitantly optimistic" at Miriam's chances of survival. Considering the situation, this update was somewhat positive. It was astonishing how much our lives have changed in the last few days. Miriam was still knocking on heaven's door and luckily there had not yet been an answer.

After a few minutes of quiet reflection Bill took Sara and Jessica aside. The three of them stood in a tight circle embracing one other. Bill told them that the family needed to be strong, and that they needed to come to terms with the possibility that Miriam may not come back to them as the same person she had been. Regardless, they would accept their mother however she came home, if she came home. These were heavy words for an excruciatingly difficult time.

As I sat watching Sara, Jessica and Bill, I imagined Miriam's funeral. I envisioned Saint Nicholas Church, the flowers, the mourners, the casket. I was not sure how the family would be able to survive such a sad and horrible event. Also, I started to contemplate what life would be like without Miriam. How would Bill cope? How would Sara and Jessica cope? Sammy would not know his grandmother. This was very similar to my situation and my mom's mother. She died when I was around Sammy's age – too young to lose a grandparent.

At this desperate and dark moment I wanted to do something helpful so I made a deal with God. I said in my heart to God that if He allowed Miriam to live and make it home, in any way, shape, or form, I would be a better person and live my life in a way that I would help others. I meant this with all my heart and soul. Time would tell if God would answer my prayer and accept this deal. The song "Unanswered Prayers" by Garth Brooks kept entering my mind. The song's titular line is "Some of God's greatest gifts are unanswered prayers." I hoped my prayer, however, was answered.

There was a high probability that Miriam could die at any moment or remain in a vegetative and unresponsive state for the rest of her days. The family was coming to terms with this reality. We also knew that Miriam was tough and chances were she was fighting like hell inside her small, beaten down frame. We were certain she was attempting to wake up and we were hoping that she had the strength and wherewithal to succeed. No one knows for certain what occurs in a person's brain when they are in a coma, but I like to think that Miriam was doing what she could to make herself wake up and beat the odds that were stacking more and more against her like unbearable weights being added to a bending barbell.

As this long day was winding down it was reported to us by one of the nurses that Miriam might have shrugged her shoulders slightly and might have moved a few fingers and toes. *Might* was the critical word. Promising news to end this day, but not enough to instill happiness or relief. The nurse was not sure if these were involuntary or voluntary movements or if she saw them at all.

We had dinner at Jessica and James's home that night. After dinner I drove Sara, Bill and Jessica to the hospital to say goodnight to Miriam. I waited outside the room.

# Friday June 24th

*"I don't think of all the misery but of the beauty that still remains."*
*-Anne Frank*

Friday was another trying day. We woke up slowly, and after picking beans and other scrumptious vegetables, Sara and I dropped Mandy off with my mom. She was always asking what she could do to help. Taking Mandy was extremely helpful. Sara and I drove to the hospital.

The first thing we learned when we arrived at the hospital was that the doctors had taken a sample of the fluid around Miriam's lungs. The fluid was not blood but normal, clear, bodily fluid. My dad called it seepage and he described it as the clear fluid that occurs when you get a small cut on your finger or around a hangnail. If the fluid was blood then this would suggest that there may be additional internal bleeding or that the body was not able to absorb blood properly. It was significantly more positive news that it was normal fluid. The doctors were planning on draining as much of the fluid as they could the next day.

We also learned that one of the doctors who analyzed at the CT scan from the day before suggested that there may be brain damage.

There was a dark spot in the scan that looked abnormal. This same doctor said that the spot he noticed might be old, meaning the brain had this mark on it before the cancer and it would not cause any complications, or it could be something else or nothing at all. Most of the doctors agreed that Miriam did not have brain damage, but none of them were entirely sure enough to make a definitive diagnosis. Only time would tell.

Miriam was returned to the ICU from the lower level where she had been since she was abruptly moved a few days prior. My dad and Bill ensured that the nurses and doctors knew how to notify Bill if Miriam were to be moved again. Also, the doctors reported that Miriam seemed agitated by the breathing tube. This was encouraging. She was given medication to make her more comfortable. The breathing tube creating discomfort indicated that she might be waking up and had developed sensation in her throat and esophagus. The more agitated Miriam became, the better. This might sound counter-intuitive or cruel, but the more stimuli she reacted to indicated that she might be waking up from the coma, but it was difficult to determine.

We left the hospital after eating lunch at the Bing Dining Room. I had the familiar and consistent club sandwich with skinny fries. I dropped Sara off at Rancho Shopping Center where she had a deep tissue massage. The massage would hopefully help ease some of the intense stress she was under. During her massage I went to my parents' house. My mom was home with Mandy, and we took Mandy for a walk to a nearby Bank of America. On the way back we saw one of my mom's friends, Alice. Alice was a native New Yorker and like many native New Yorkers, she sure could talk. We chatted for a while, and I was getting a little nervous about being late to pick up Sara as the friend carried on.

After the walk I picked up Sara from her massage. I arrived just as she was finishing, then we went to the hospital. There was not any new information and Miriam's condition had not changed. We went to dinner at Jessica and James's where we had soup. We talked about the next evening when we would be participating in a Relay For Life at the Los Altos High School track. We also watched the cross bay rivals, the Oakland Athletics and the San Francisco Giants, play each other in baseball on the television. I don't recall who won.

Later that evening I drove Sara, Bill and Jessica to the hospital to say goodnight to Miriam. This time, instead of parking the car in the parking garage and all of us going into the hospital, I parked the car in front of the hospital on the street and waited in the idling car while they went inside to say goodnight and check on her condition. Waiting in the car gave me time to reflect on what had happened so far. The definitive conclusion that I could make at this point was that cancer really is a horrible monster that needs to be eradicated.

# Saturday June 25th

*"The word 'happiness' would lose its meaning if it were not balanced by sadness." -Carl Gustav Jung*

We woke up and met at the hospital. Miriam had another CT scan. The doctors wanted to take another look at her brain. Since she had still not wakened it was becoming more and more frightening and pointing towards brain damage or brain injury. Once the doctors got the results of the tests back they were fairly certain that there was no brain damage. This was a huge relief.

However, with something positive came something negative. We also learned that Miriam's right leg was in extremely bad condition. The toes were purple and bruised and the entire leg was grotesquely swollen. Her leg was swollen much worse than her arm had been. The doctors said that they would perform a blood clot scope to see if they could locate the clot and hopefully clear it and save the leg. A blood clot scope was more intrusive and dangerous than an ultrasound. But since the leg was larger than the arm and had larger veins and arteries, the doctors thought the scope might tell them more about the blood clot. They were not sure when they would perform this procedure but there was a high probability that Miriam would lose a foot and possibly part of her leg because of the clot.

We also learned that the fluid around Miriam's lungs was drained. The doctors removed nearly a quart of clear liquid. A quart is thirty-two ounces and weights approximately 2.15 pounds. This was much more liquid than any of the doctors hypothesized they would collect. I imagine the liquid was extracted with a large syringe but I did not ask.

With the fluid gone, some of the doctors' hypothesis was that Miriam would be able to breathe easier and get her lungs working more efficiently. Having thirty-two ounces of pressure around her lungs probably impeded her breathing and helped keep her in the coma. Also, the doctors told us that her eyes almost looked normal. However, she was still not waking up from the sedation and did not respond to stimuli. It was positive that her eyes were looking healthier than they had in the past.

The last bit of news that the doctors shared with us was that her liver did not seem damaged. This was very positive. Removing the fluid around her lungs might also have helped the liver. We spent the rest of the afternoon waiting, praying, walking and drinking water. Everyone really missed Miriam.

We had dinner with my mom and dad at Jessica and James's house. My mom prepared shrimp skewers which were tasty. Once dinner ended, Sara and I drove to Los Altos High School to participate in the Relay For Life.

Relay For Life is an event designed to celebrate cancer survivorship, remember its victims and raise awareness and funds for cancer research and American Cancer Society programs. During the twenty-four hour event, teams of people gather at schools, fairgrounds, or parks and take turns walking or running laps around a track. Each team tried to keep at least one member on the track at all times during the twenty-four hours. Since cancer is awake twenty four hours a day, so should someone from a team.

This was the first year that the Relay For Life was being held at Los Altos High School. Ironically, Bill and Miriam had actively supported this wonderful event before it was known that Miriam had cancer. Relay For Life events take place around the world.

Jessica, James, Bill and one of Bill's neighbors, Todd, met Sara and me at the track. Sara and I arrived first and we went to the sign-in tent. Two ladies greeted us and asked if we'd signed in yet. We said no and they gave us a waiver to sign stating that we could not sue if we got hurt at the event. We signed and looked around for someone familiar.

We found the area where all the team tents were pitched. Teams erected campsites for the twenty-four hour event. Some participants slept over while others congregated at the team site during the event when they were not walking on the track. Some teams were very creative and developed elaborate sites and themes. Most of the themes were cancer orientated. Examples of themes could be teams that try to raise awareness about various cancers, provide information on services for cancer patients, plus other cancer-oriented ideas. A campsite I saw at a recent Relay For Life was a takeoff of the television show *Survivor*. The relay team was called Survivor Ovarian. They created their campsite in a beach survivor theme and educated others about ovarian cancer. They designed t-shirts, flags, and other intricate props.

Sara and I could not locate a tent for Team Maltby's, which was a local restaurant in Los Altos and the team for which we were walking. We walked around the other campsites and decided to head back toward the track. As we were searching, we found Jessica and James and then saw Bill. We began to walk the track together at eight in the evening. Dozens of friends joined us in the walk while the sun was setting. This was a very emotional moment for the family as these friends had been praying for and supporting all of us and Miriam in her battle. Bill had hats made with Miriam's name on them. We wore these with pride and conviction.

Along the inside and outside border of the track were luminaries, decorated paper bags which contained a light source, usually a glow stick or a small candle. Luminaries were similar to Chinese paper lanterns. Each was decorated in honor of someone who had survived cancer, was battling cancer, or had lost the fight to cancer. I saw numerous luminaries with Miriam's name and messages of hope and perseverance on them while we continued to walk.

As we walked we saw quite a few people we knew and many more that we did not. The feeling around the track was one of unity and perseverance. There was a section of the track that had a stage and featured a variety of speakers and entertainment. As we were walking, a young lady on the stage was describing how she'd learned she had cancer before her wedding. She got married and then fought for her life against the cancer. She was now pregnant and cancer free. There were other speakers also sharing their stories as we walked.

As the sun was setting the luminaries began to glow brightly. At one point the master of ceremonies requested that all cancer survivors form a chain on the track by holding a paper chain link between each person. This human chain of cancer survivors covered three-fourths of the track. The human chain crept slowly around the track as everyone watched. This was extremely emotional and moving.

This walk taught me that cancer affects many people and needs to be eradicated. Hopefully, someday soon it will be.

Once our hour of walking came to an end and the sun disappeared into the west, we prepared to leave the track. The luminaries were glowing brightly in the clear night sky. I said a quick prayer for Miriam and for everyone touched by cancer. We got in our cars and went home.

# Sunday June 26th

*"Do not be afraid of tomorrow; for God is already there." (Author Unknown)*

We awoke Sunday morning and I watered the garden and picked more of the ever abundant green beans. They grow aggressively! After that I took a shower, ate breakfast, and went to mass. Later in the afternoon Father Gary was giving his last mass at Saint Nicholas before his sabbatical and reassignment, which would lead him to the Vatican where he would train to be an exorcist. The mass we attended at 10am was given by Father Larry. It was uplifting and allowed time for all of us to pray and to reflect upon what was happening.

After mass, Sara and I went to a local bakery and restaurant called Le Boulanger where we both ate a breakfast sandwich. From there we went to the hospital.

At the hospital we had a pleasant conversation with Doctor Jamieson. Doctor Jamieson was one of the doctors who had been caring for Miriam while she was in the ICU. During this talk the doctor covered the issues concerning Miriam's condition and progress. The first issue was that Miriam was still not waking up, which was the most urgent and worrisome. One theory was that she had an infection that was stopping her from waking. The doctors were going to administer an MRI later that day or the next to determine Miriam's brain activity and why she was not waking.

An MRI (Magnetic Resonance Imaging) is a non-invasive method used to render images of the inside of an object. It is primarily used in medicine to demonstrate pathological or other physiological alterations of living tissues. MRI provides an unparalleled view inside the human body. The level of detail that can be seen is extraordinary compared with any other imaging modality. MRI is the method of choice for the diagnosis of many types of injuries and conditions because of the incredible ability to tailor the exam to the particular medical question being asked. By changing exam parameters, the MRI system can cause tissues in the body to take on different appearances. This is especially helpful to a radiologist in determining if something seen is normal. One of the reasons Miriam did not have an MRI earlier was because the scanners can cost over three million dollars each and cost several hundred thousand dollars per year to maintain. MRI scanners are used sparingly because of these extreme costs.

The second issue, which was positive, was that Miriam's breathing was improving. She was on fifty percent oxygen versus one hundred percent oxygen the day before. But, as we learned over the past few days, the oxygen percentage fluctuated greatly and did not really indicate significant progress unless it consistently stayed at a low level for a long period of time. The third issue was that the fluid did not return to the area around her lungs. This was great news and could also be related to her improved breathing.

During this conversation with Doctor Jamieson my dad asked a question that James's mom asked my dad. The question was,

"Would all of these complications have happened if Miriam started chemotherapy a day later than she did?"

Doctor Jamieson's answer was, "These complications might not have happened but Miriam probably would have died if she did not begin chemotherapy when she did. Her cancer was quite aggressive and waiting a day longer might have been a day too late. The cancer would have probably spread to her heart."

This answer was honest and to the point. Thank goodness Miriam was at Stanford Hospital. These doctors were miracle workers.

Sara, my dad and I walked to a nearby market called Andronico's where we got sandwiches for lunch. It was therapeutic to get out of the hospital and take a walk.

Later that day two of my friends, John and Amanda, visited. I've known John since junior high. We share the same birthday, were in Boy Scouts together and were also in each other's weddings. Sara, John, Amanda and I took a long walk around the Stanford University campus. It was a hot and dry day. Stanford has a fairly large campus with more than 46 miles of roads, a 49-megawatt power plant, two separate water systems, three dams and lakes, 78 miles of water mains, a central heating and cooling plant, a high-voltage distribution system and a post office. The university is a self-sustaining community. Stanford also provides or contracts for its own fire, police and other services.

There are more than 670 major buildings at Stanford that incorporate 13.1 million square feet. Ninety-five percent of undergraduates live on campus, as do nearly sixty percent of graduate students and thirty percent of faculty members. There are 850 owner-occupied housing units and 628 rental units for faculty and staff. Stanford is one of the most energy efficient institutions among California research universities. The campus cogeneration plant produces all the energy the campus needs, plus an extra twenty megawatts at peak that is provided for public consumption. Stanford recycles more than half the waste generated on campus.

There are also over 43,000 trees on the Stanford campus with the Coast Live Oak being the most common. Stanford's current mascot is a student dressed in a tree costume. Many of Stanford's picturesque redwoods, cedars, Canary Island palms and eucalyptus trees have survived a century or more of drought, flood and change. There are more than 800 different species of plants on campus. The inner campus includes more than 1.4 million square feet of shrubs, 190,000 linear feet of groundcovers, 1.2 million square feet of lawns and 2,300 automatic irrigation valves. There are 16 fountains.

Life outside the hospital was progressing as usual. People were bustling about, moving from one place to the next. There were bridal parties and Quinceañeras taking pictures in front of the beautiful and picturesque Stanford Memorial Church. We walked past Hoover Tower and through a few of the campus sculpture gardens.

Stanford Memorial Church is the dominant architectural feature of the Main Quadrangle on the campus. Memorial Church was dedicated in 1903 in memory of Leland Stanford. Memorial Church has been non-sectarian since its inception. One especially striking feature of the church is the brilliant mosaic covering the interior walls and depicting scenes from the Hebrew Bible. The stained glass windows depict scenes from the New Testament. The church features nearly 20,000 shades of color in the tile mosaics, thirty-four shades of pink alone in the cheeks of the four angels in the dome.

Memorial Church features four organs, including the Fisk-Nanney organ, which has 73 ranks and 4,332 pipes. It is quite a sight.

Hoover Tower, like Memorial Church, draws a gaggle of visitors and is visible from almost every part of the campus. This 285-foot landmark offers views of campus, the foothills and the Santa Clara Valley. The Lou Henry and Herbert Hoover rooms contain documents and memorabilia from the Hoovers' lives and travels. To date, Herbert Hoover is the only President of the United States who graduated from Stanford University.

The Campus Sculpture Garden contains an extensive collection of outdoor art located throughout campus. Among more than seventy sculptures are works by Auguste Rodin, Henry Moore, Josef Albers, Alexander Calder, George Segal and Joan Miró. Stone River by Andy Goldsworthy, Miwok by Mark di Suvero and Three Sentinels by Beverly Pepper are among the newest sculptures on campus. The Papua New Guinea Sculpture Garden features the carving methods, cultural traditions and mythological heritage of the Kwoma and Iatmul people of Papua New Guinea. The B. Gerald Cantor Rodin Sculpture Garden contains more than twenty works by Auguste Rodin, including The Gates of Hell. Stanford is beautiful.

After our walk, John and Amanda lingered for a little while longer and then they left. We had a pleasant visit and they were very supportive. It was refreshing to see and experience the outside world.

For dinner that night we went to James and Jessica's house and had barbecued pork ribs. I believe James's parents joined us.

After dinner, Sara, Bill, Jessica and I went to the hospital to visit Miriam. I parked the car and we all went in to see her. The nurse she had was pleasant and positive and Miriam looked better than she did the last time I saw her, which was fantastic.

After leaving the hospital, Sara and I went to my parents' house. We visited with my parents and my siblings. It was positive to be with family. After that we went back to Sara's parents' house and retired for the night.

# Monday June 27th

*"God puts rainbows in the clouds so that each of us – in the dreariest and most dreaded moments – can see a possibility of hope. -Maya Angelou*

This was the twenty-sixth day since the initial X-ray that showed the cancerous mass of tissue in Miriam. This day, like many before, would become sad and worrisome. Sara and I got up and after picking vegetables and watering the garden we made our way to the hospital to meet Bill.

When we arrived at the hospital we learned that there had been trouble with one of Miriam's nurses. This was a different nurse than the night before. The nurse would not allow Bill to see Miriam in the morning and she was very nasty and rude. Bill called my dad, who came over immediately.

The nurse was rude to him also. Dad acted fast and spoke to the head nurse and others at the hospital. Bill also spoke to some people. We were assured that the situation was resolved and that this mean-spirited nurse would not be caring for Miriam again.

It turned out that the nurse was leaving Stanford and probably had a record of poor people skills. This demonstrated that even a great hospital like Stanford has its share of problems.

The primary issues for this day were that Miriam was not waking up and that she had a fever. One theory was that she could have an infection or virus (maybe meningitis or herpes) that was not allowing her to wake. The fever suggested that she was fighting an infection. This was a new and potentially deadly complication.

The doctors planned to perform a spinal tap later that day or in the morning the next day where they would look for signs of meningitis or herpes. A spinal tap is also known as a lumbar puncture. It is a diagnostic, and at times therapeutic, procedure that is performed in order to collect a sample of cerebrospinal fluid for biochemical, microbiological, and cytological analysis, or to relieve increased intracranial pressure.

The most common purpose for a lumbar puncture is to collect cerebrospinal fluid in a case of suspected meningitis, since there is no other reliable tool with which meningitis can be excluded and it is often a life-threatening but highly treatable condition. Infants commonly require lumbar puncture as a part of the routine workup for fever without a source, as they have a much higher risk of meningitis than older persons and do not reliably show signs of meningeal irritation (meningismus).

Lumbar punctures may also be done to inject medications into the cerebrospinal fluid, particularly for spinal anesthesia or chemotherapy. A lumbar puncture requires that the skin that will be punctured be sterile, and it must be performed by qualified and skilled medical practitioners. Spinal needles are used in lumbar puncture.

When performing a lumbar puncture, first the patient is placed in a left or right lateral position with his or her neck bent in full flexion and knees bent in full flexion up to his or her chest, approximating a fetal position as much as possible. The area around the lower back is prepared using aseptic technique. Once the appropriate location is palpated, local anesthetic is infiltrated under the skin and then injected along the intended path of the spinal needle. A spinal needle is inserted between the lumbar vertebrae L3/L4 or L4/L5 and pushed in until there is a "give." The "give" indicates the needle is past the dura mater. The stylet from the spinal needle is then withdrawn and drops of cerebrospinal fluid are collected. The fluid is useful in determining if the patient has contracted meningitis.

We ate lunch at the Bing Dining Room and were informed that we could no longer pay for meals as long as we were still in the hospital. Our meals were being "taken care of" by the hospital, which was extremely gracious. We had become a fixture.

Also at the Bing, we had the same waiter each day for lunch. His name was Kit and he was hard working, always smiling and extremely pleasant. He told us that he did not necessarily like working at the restaurant but he was good to talk to and provided excellent service. Kit is an example of one of the usually anonymous hospital employees that we came to know.

Later that day my mom visited us at the hospital. Bill was asleep on one of the couches so my mom and I took a walk around the Stanford campus. It was good to walk and talk with her. She showed me many parts of the campus that I did not know existed.

Later that evening we went to James and Jessica's' house for dinner where we had pork chops. After dinner I took Sara, Jessica and Bill to the hospital to say goodnight to Miriam. I waited in the idling car.

# Tuesday June 28th

*"Life is a shipwreck but we must not forget to sing in the lifeboats." -Voltaire*

After waking, watering the garden, and having a quick breakfast, Sara and I headed to the hospital. We saw Miriam and her eyes were partway open! They had been closed when we saw her last. I could see the white of her eyes and half of her pupil. Her eyes were not focused and they looked extremely fatigued and dazed. I could not tell if she actually saw us. If she did, she did not react. She did have a great nurse, named Madonna, who was extremely warm and caring. It was comforting to know Miriam was being cared for.

We went back to the waiting room and met Jessica and Sammy. I saw Sammy fuss for the first time ever. It looked like he was having a bad day. Later that afternoon, Jessica, Bill, and Sara visited Miriam. They said she acknowledged them with a shifting of her eyes. This was fantastic and was the most hopeful breakthrough yet! The mood for the rest of the day and evening was positive and upbeat. Also, the result of the spinal tap came back and there were no indications of meningitis. Miriam's fever was dissipating. This was extremely positive and welcome news. I was not sure if this officially meant she was out of the coma, but it really did not matter. We were not ready to declare victory because Miriam's life was still in immediate danger, but the dark cloud surrounding us seemed to be dissolving a smidgen.

In the afternoon I stopped by my parent's house. My mom had baked a hug tray of cookies for the ICU nurses, doctors and staff. The tray was so large that I had a difficult time holding it and keeping it level. I delivered the cookies to the ICU and, as luck would have it, the nurse Madonna was on her break outside of Miriam's room. I handed her the tray of cookies. She was very grateful. I am sure the nurses, doctors and staff enjoyed the delicious snacks. In most workplaces, if the two words "free" and "food" are combined, the free edible items usually disappear quickly. It was also a good idea to make friends with the ICU nurses. Cookies have been known to create and build countless friendships over the years. I bet they could stop wars.

I do not recall what we ate for lunch but I imagine we went to the Bing. I also do not recall what we did for dinner that night. I do know that I drove Sara, Bill and Jessica to the hospital after dinner so they could say goodnight to Miriam. She was moving slightly but was still bedridden and did not know what was occurring. It was comforting not to have a whole lot to say on this day. In this situation, no news was definitely good news.

# Wednesday June 29th

*"Courage and perseverance have a magical talisman, before which difficulties disappear and obstacles vanish into air." -John Quincy Adams*

Sara and I pulled away from her parents' house at 8am in our Ford Explorer. We were driving south to Los Angeles and aiming to arrive before the start of afternoon L.A. gridlock. The trip from Sara's parents' home to El Segundo is approximately four hundred miles. I would be happy if we arrived in El Segundo by four-thirty that afternoon. Before we got on the road we purchased two sandwiches and some water from a local grocery store.

We made great time the first two hundred miles. The traffic was light and the day was beautiful. We stopped at a rest stop five miles before the halfway point between Los Angeles and San Jose in the agriculture-heavy San Joaquin Valley to go to the bathroom and stretch our legs. After the quick stop we continued south on Interstate 5.

I was driving around eighty-five miles per hour in the right lane on the two lane highway. I moved to the left lane and accelerated to pass a slower moving truck. As my foot pressed down on the accelerator the Explorer lost all power. The gas pedal went limp and the car was losing speed fast. All I could do was coast to a stop on the narrow left lane shoulder and hope another vehicle did not clip us from behind.

As the Explorer came to a stop on the left side of the interstate my mind was racing as what to do next. I turned off the ignition and then turned it back on. The car made a faint sputtering noise and the low oil warning light illuminated, then nothing. The car would not start. I did this a few more times with the same result. Meanwhile, with the car stopped on the left side of the road, trucks, buses and cars were zooming past us barely a few feet from hitting us. This was not the place to breakdown.

To the left of us was long, brittle, golden tinted grass and a small hill. Beyond the hill was the freeway going north in the opposite direction. Luckily we did not breakdown on a true median where there was barely any room between the swiftly moving north and south traffic.

Sara called AAA as we were beginning to bake in the hot car. The temperature outside was in the low nineties and the temperature inside felt like an oven. AAA said a tow truck should be there in forty-five minutes or less. We had to wait.

I made the decision that we should wait outside of the car rather than in it, figuring that if someone hit the car while we were inside then we could be seriously injured. Also, it was getting very hot in the car.

We waited approximately fifteen feet from the car in the dry grass. The area we were in contained brittle, golden grass, tumbleweed and I am sure a few families of snakes. The grass was about waist high and razor sharp. As we stood and waited I tried not to make any sudden movements and kept my eyes moving, scanning for snakes or other creatures with fangs, venom or sharp teeth. I noticed to the left of us up on a hill there were two large holes dug into the earth. I imagined a family of hungry coyotes emerging and seeing us as an easy midday snack. I decided not to share my fears or observations with Sara. It turned out that she also had the same fears and did not want to share them with me.

As we waited I could feel the sun baking my skin. I did not apply sunscreen and was wearing shorts and a short sleeve shirt. Sara was also baking. She was both better off and worse off than me. She was better off because she was wearing jeans. The jeans protected her legs from the sharp grass, menacing tumbleweeds, and relentless thorns. She was worse off because she was not wearing substantial shoes but thin sandals. As I stood in the grass I prayed for Miriam, for snakes to keep away, and that somehow we make it home by the end of the day.

A tow truck eventually arrived. The driver pulled in front of our car and exited the cab. He was a middle-aged man who walked bowlegged and said very few words. He asked if the car could move. I was tempted to respond, "If the car could move then why did we call you?" But instead I said, "No, it does not start." Without looking at me, or trying to start the car, he began the tedious and frightening task of lifting our Explorer onto the bed of the tow truck while cars and trucks were flying past at high speeds. Somehow our vehicle made it on.

Sara and I joined the driver in the cab of his dirty and well worn truck that looked like he lived in it. Once we got in the truck the driver asked us where we wanted to go. I said Kettleman City since it was only one mile away and the only place I knew around the area. We usually stopped for gas in Kettleman City. He did not say a word but put the tow truck in gear and began to rumble down the interstate.

Kettleman City's population was 1,499 at the 2000 census. It is near the halfway point between Los Angeles and San Francisco or Sacramento on Interstate 5. It is a major stopping point for food and gasoline. Kettleman City is also near a large 1,600-acre hazardous waste and municipal solid waste disposal facility.

Once we were in Kettleman City I asked the driver, whose name I believe was Joshua, which mechanic he recommended. He was quiet for a few moments and then replied by saying that there was only one mechanic in Kettleman City, and he hardly worked at all. I didn't know what to say to this, so I said nothing. I was starting to get scared. Why would this person take us to a place without a mechanic? I tried to keep my cool.

Joshua drove us past Kettleman City and turned left. He drove through a worn-looking truck stop that was closed and had uneven boards over its broken windows. He then turned into a worse looking trailer park that looked deserted. It consisted of off-white, sun bleached, dirty trailers spread out randomly on a flat dirt field. The trailer park looked like it had been there for quite a while and was in disrepair. I did not notice any signs of life among the scattered trailers.

As the truck rumbled and bumped through the trailer park I was not sure what was happening. Was this man going to take us somewhere to rob us or worse? Was he going to leave our car in a trailer park and take off? My mind was racing. Eventually Joshua stopped the truck in front of one of the trailers. There was a red pickup truck parked in front of it that did not have any tires and was on blocks. Joshua got out, walked to the trailer, and pounded on the door with his closed right fist. I felt relieved because I was guessing that the only mechanic in town must live in this trailer. But I was frightened about what this person might look like and what was going to happen next. I felt like I was in a horror movie where Sara and I were the unfortunate people who were the first victims at the beginning of the film.

No one seemed to be home. I was not sure if this was positive or negative. Joshua got back in the truck. I asked him where the closest mechanic was. Joshua replied, "Avenal." We were on our way to Avenal, wherever that was.

Avenal is a city in Kings County, California. It is part of the Hanford-Corcoran Metropolitan Statistical Area which encompasses all of Kings County. The population was 15,689 at the 2000 census. 7,062 of these residents were inmates at the all male Avenal State Prison. The prison was built in 1987 to accommodate 2,320 inmates. Prison overpopulation is a major problem in California. Many of the remaining Avenal residents either work at the prison, in the local agriculture industry, or did not work at all. The prison provides approximately 1,000 jobs. The city's motto is "Oasis in the Sun." Avenal is located about fifteen miles north of Kettleman City and five miles west of highway 5.

The road to Avenal was actually quite scenic. The town lies in a sun kissed valley surrounded by rolling fields. On our way to the town, Joshua picked up his cell phone and made a call.

"What are you doing?" inquired Joshua to the person on the other end.

Joshua listened for a few seconds and then said, "Well, I've got a present for you. Christmas is comin' early this year." Joshua said this in a sinister tone of voice which made me feel uncomfortable. It was clear that Sara, the car, and I were the "present" of which he spoke.

"Be there in ten minutes," snorted Joshua as he ended the phone call.

As we approached the town of Avenal I felt uneasy. I was not sure what we were in for. As the tow truck lumbered its way down the main street I scanned the buildings for a hotel or somewhere we could stay if needed. I did not see a hotel or anything welcoming. I also looked for a police station, but did not see one. The town was dirty, sun burned and worn-out. All I saw were old, depressed buildings and people looking at us suspiciously. I assumed that it was not every day that a new Ford Explorer was paraded down this sad and forgotten road in this sad and forgotten town. Finally, the tow truck pulled into a service station called "The Oasis."

An oasis it was not. There were four garages in front of us and a number of vehicles in various states of disrepair strewn around the fenced lot. The lot was enclosed by a rusting ten foot wrought iron fence. I was not sure if the fence was to keep people in or keep them out. Joshua unhooked our car and gave us the bill. It was $40 for the tow. I thought AAA offered free towing but I was not in a position to argue. I later found out that AAA paid for the first seven miles of a tow. The bill was accurate. We paid the bill with a credit card. This made Joshua perturbed because he had to call in the charge on his phone. He clearly preferred cash.

Regardless, we were in the middle of nowhere, our car would not start, and I was beginning to panic. We had approximately five hours of daylight remaining.

One of the mechanics, who rode into The Oasis on a bicycle, walked up to Joshua. I guessed this was who he was talking to on the cell phone. Joshua and the mechanic were whispering, pointing at us and the car, and whispering some more.

The mechanic, who was probably my age or a little older, walked up to me. I explained the situation. He called over a few other men in Spanish. They pushed our car into one of the garages after moving the car that was in that garage out of the way.

They opened the hood of the Explorer and had a powwow around it. Sara and I took a seat on two dirty plastic chairs that were in the garage. We slowly ate the sandwiches we'd brought from Los Altos.

After ten minutes the mechanic came over to us. He said it would cost $125 for him to look at the car and that they only accept cash. He also said that the only ATM in town was owned by The Oasis and was in a far corner of the junk yard. Convenient, I thought.

Luckily Sara and I had about $140 dollars cash between us. I agreed to the estimate and signed the estimate paper.

I watched the mechanics as they worked. They stood around the engine as one of them tried to start the car. The car did not start. They took tools and poked a few things. Still no good.

Five minutes later the mechanic told me that they were not sure what was wrong with the car. He said that Ford did not release their diagnostic tools to the general public until a few years after a certain car model was released. Since we had a new Explorer they did not have the proper tools to diagnose the problem. As the mechanic was telling me this my mind was racing. What would we do? Sleep in the car? Tow it to the closest Ford dealership? That could be hundreds of miles away. The mechanic said he would do what he could. He walked back to the car.

About ten minutes later the mechanics were excited. They discovered the source of the problem without the diagnostic tools. One of the cables to the battery had come undone. They plugged it back in and started the car. We were charged $80 for the fix.

I gladly handed the mechanic a one hundred dollar bill. He walked over to a tackle box looking for change. The box was full of about twenty one hundred dollar bills, but there was not any change. He closed the tackle box and walked over to a group of guys standing on the sidewalk with our one hundred dollars. The group talked for a few moments, pointed at Sara and me, did some sort of transaction, and then the mechanic walked back to me. He handed me a twenty dollar bill. I got in the Explorer, turned it on, thanked the mechanic, and we were on our way out of Avenal, back on the road.

I said a silent prayer of thanks as we drove from Avenal. We got back on highway 5 south and headed toward El Segundo.

Relieved, we eventually arrived, unloaded our gear and went to the park for the Round Robin tennis class. We did not play but made sure that everyone had plenty of tennis balls and knew what they were going to do. After the class was situated we got food, went home and went to bed. What a day.

# Thursday June 30th

*"Healing takes courage, and we all have courage, even if we have to dig a little to find it."* -Tori Amos

I spent the next morning at a Ford dealership service center. I thought it would be prudent if they examined the car. The mechanics at the dealership seemed genuinely concerned with what had happened and four hours later I was on my way. They did not provide a reason why the cable came undone but they assured me that they sealed it on extremely well.

After the dealership I drove to the carwash and washed the car. I next went home and did the same to some dirty laundry.

That night, Sara and I ate Mexican food for dinner at a restaurant called Haciendas where I ate too much. We had been going to Haciendas for years. It was a comfortable place near El Segundo and Loyola Marymount University that made us feel at home. We still patronize this restaurant when we can. When a certain waiter, named Ezekiel, sees us, he immediately prepares a pitcher of margaritas on the rocks without us even needing to ask for it. That's service and hospitality at its finest.

# Friday July 1st

*"Our sorrows and wounds are healed only when we touch them with compassion." -Buddha*

We woke up early and a neighbor drove us to LAX. This was becoming an all too familiar routine. Once we arrived in San Jose we were picked up and went to visit Miriam. When I walked into her room in the ICU I noticed a significant improvement. She was not talking or moving but her color looked better and there were fewer machines in the room and not as many tubes attached to her body. She even opened her eyes from time to time. This was promising. I do not believe she knew we were there necessarily, nor was she able to control her eye movement.

She was nearing the two week mark in ICU. Once someone is in the ICU for more than two weeks and on a breathing apparatus during that time, it is common to consider long term options, and difficult decisions are often made. The ICU is for someone who has an emergency issue and requires constant care. Once the issue is resolved, digresses, does not change, or the patient dies, they will leave the ICU. The doctors were looking at options such as transferring Miriam to a hospice, being able to send her home with a good deal of assistance, and other possibilities. It was a sad fact that her ICU room was needed by other people with more need than Miriam.

The doctors were starting to talk about the possibility of having to perform a tracheotomy if Miriam did not fully wake up and breathe on her own. This is a serious procedure and would severely delay any recovery. However, having this done would make it possible for Miriam to transfer out of the ICU because she would not be reliant on the machines to help her breathe. These machines were not portable.

A tracheotomy is a surgical procedure in which a cut or opening is made in the trachea, also known as the windpipe. The surgeon inserts a tube into the opening to bypass an obstruction, allowing air to get to the lungs. The term tracheostomy is sometimes used interchangeably with tracheotomy. Strictly speaking, however, tracheostomy usually refers to the opening itself while a tracheotomy is the procedure.

A tracheotomy is performed if ample oxygen is not getting to the lungs, if the person cannot breathe without help, or is having problems with mucus and other secretions getting into the windpipe because of difficulty swallowing. There are many reasons why air cannot get to the lungs. The patient's windpipe may be blocked by a swelling; by a severe injury to the neck, nose or mouth; by a large foreign object; by paralysis of the throat muscles; or by a tumor. The patient may be in a coma or need a ventilator to pump air into the lungs for a long period of time. Doctors perform tracheotomies as last-resort procedures. They are done only if the patient's windpipe is obstructed and the situation is life-threatening. This was a procedure none of us wanted to see Miriam subjected to.

Also, Sara had a cold she was fighting. She diligently donned a surgical mask that covered her mouth and nose when visiting her mother and constantly applied hand sanitizer. Sara and I also decided that we were not going on the Lane family vacation later in the summer, because we did not want to be too far away. The rest of my family was going on a weeklong cruise to Mexico.

The remainder of the day was spent at the hospital. We hoped that Miriam would fully wake up so that she did not have to have the tracheotomy. This was another long and difficult day.

# Saturday July 2nd

*"It's not the years in your life that count. It's the life in your years."*
*-Abraham Lincoln*

I woke up Sunday morning around seven after not sleeping well. I had been tormenting myself about how to inform my mom that Sara and I were not going on the family cruise. I knew that Sara was correct and that we should not go, but I also knew that my mom had put a great deal of energy and money into the event.

After breakfast I picked up the phone and called my parents. My dad answered. I told him that we'd decided that Sara and I would not be going on the cruise. He told me that he agreed with my decision and that he was going to speak to me about not going on the cruise later that day. I'd beat him to the punch.

As I hung up the phone I felt much better.

I showered and got ready to go to the hospital.

Today turned out to be a positive day considering the circumstances. Miriam's breathing had improved significantly. It was so good that her breathing tube had been removed. There was no more talk about a tracheotomy. Miriam could also make audible sounds and her eyes were wide open. It looked like she was waking!

My mom visited us at the hospital, and I asked her if dad told her that I would not be going on the cruise. She said he did and that was the end of the conversation.

Bill had become accustomed to taking his afternoon naps on a couch in the waiting area or somewhere else in the hospital. Today was no exception. But today he was much happier than usual and had an aura about him that suggested extra energy that had no outlet. For the first time in who knows how long, all of his, and our, energy was not focused on Miriam and her struggles for survival because she was doing so well. We all, especially Bill, seemed happy. This was fantastic.

The catalyst, according to the nurse, that helped Miriam start to wake up from her coma was the Food Network. Whenever the Food Network was turned on the nurse noticed that Miriam became more agitated and tried to move. She almost seemed angry. This agitation and activity was the best thing for her. Because of this action her body was forced to respond and create more stimuli. Miriam enjoyed cooking and watching the Food Network. She could have possibly heard the program and wanted desperately to see it as well. Also, there was a picture of Sammy placed on the wall at the end of her bed. This photograph was always in Miriam's line of vision. If she saw this picture I am sure it made her fight harder to wake up from the coma. She did not want to die and miss out on spending time with her grandchild.

One hurdle that still needed to be overcome before Miriam could leave the ICU was that her PICC line needed to be removed. The doctors were not yet prepared for this step. Once they were, Miriam could be transferred to a non-ICU room in the hospital. The doctors did not want to remove the PICC line because if they did, it would be difficult to administer medication quickly if it were needed. Miriam still had the feeding tube but its removal was not a prerequisite to leave the ICU. She could not feed herself. The muscles that aid in swallowing had not been used in weeks and would need to be re-taught how to function properly.

That night, Pete came over for dinner. He was a friend of the family and someone Bill had known a very long time. We had a feast of fresh salmon, grilled garden vegetables and other delectable treats. All of us pitched in to set the table, serve and cook the food, and clean. It was apparent that we did not have the meal preparation skills that Miriam possessed, but we got by well enough. We were happy that it looked like Miriam was going to get out of the ICU. We were also hopeful that she would wake up further, regain her ability to speak and regain her memory. This was a good day.

# Sunday July 3rd

*"Although the world is full of suffering, it is also full of the overcoming of it." -Helen Keller*

Sara and I woke, went to church and were met Bill, Jessica, James, Sammy, my mom and dad. I opted to sit with my parents while Sara sat with Bill, Jessica, James and Sammy. They sat in their usual place in the back of the church, while my parents and I sat in the middle.

After mass, Sara and I went to the House of Bagels, grabbed a bagel, and headed to the hospital. Today was the day that Miriam was going to be moved out of the ICU if her PICC line could be removed.

Sara and I went to see Miriam at the hospital. What a surprise! Her eyes were fully open and she looked at us when we walked in the room. My heart almost burst with joy.

She had begun to speak! Sara and I spoke with her a little. We did not know what to say. It was ludicrously ironic that we had hoped, prayed, and willed her to speak for so long and now that she could, we did not know what to say. This was truly a miracle.

We told her that we were there for her and that everyone was doing fine. She was extremely quiet. When she spoke she was very hard to hear or understand. I could tell Miriam was struggling to put together words and that her brain was working hard to make connections. She was extremely confused and not quite sure where she was and what was happening. The theory was that the sedation drugs were still affecting her memory and speech. They had not entirely worn off. It would take more time for the drugs to completely dissipate from her system, but she did recognize us.

Later that day my dad joined us in the room with Miriam. He asked her if she wanted to know what had happened to her. She said yes, she did. My dad told an abridged version of this story. He told me that we would have to tell her the same story over and over again for a while, because chances are she would forget the details right after she heard them.

My dad also told Sara and me a story about his mother and father that I had never heard before while we were in the waiting area. The story took place when he was younger. He grew up on a small farm in a rural town in Ohio called Centerville. He was one of five children, and his family was not rich and money was always tight. His father gave his mother a monthly allowance with which to buy food and other necessities for the family. Once the money was gone for the month she could not get anymore. This made Mom-Mom (my grandmother) extremely thrifty. She would not spend her allowance on items that were not essential for the family, but Pop-Pop (my grandfather) would spend foolishly from time to time. He would purchase frivolous items such as candy, junk food, and other nonessentials. When he did this he deducted what he spent from Mom-Mom's monthly allowance. This was not fair, but it was the reality. I enjoyed this family story.

Most of this day was spent in the hospital trying to determine when and where Miriam would be moved. We were also notified that her PICC line was coming out! Eventually, Sara and I left to do errands. We went to my parents' house to visit and then to a few other places. Sara called her dad and he told us that Miriam had been moved to another part of the hospital. He told us the room and floor.

Miriam was moved to the bone marrow transplant unit in Stanford Hospital, not because she needed a transplant, but because the rooms in this unit had the proper monitoring equipment and there was an available room. Patients coming out of a prolonged stay in ICU can be very confused and cannot be allowed to walk by themselves as a fall can be catastrophic. Monitoring was imperative.

The bone marrow transplant unit is a ward in the hospital that primarily contained bone marrow transplant patients. In most cases it was crucial that these individuals did not have contact with outside germs. If an infection or virus developed in a bone marrow patient, the effects could be deadly. Some family members visiting patients in this ward had to don full bodysuits and facemasks so as to not transmit germs to their loved ones or others in the area.

Sara, Jessica, Bill and I spent time in the room with Miriam for the remainder of the afternoon. It was awkward at times. We would talk to Miriam, ask a question, tell her a story, or make a comment. Her response was usually hard to hear and difficult to decipher. She would also ask us muffled or nonsensical questions. It was frustrating for us and for her.

Communication was a big issue. I could see in her eyes that she had a million questions but she could not verbalize them. We were almost to the point where one tap of her finger would mean yes and two would mean no. This was extremely frustrating for all of us, but we were beyond giddy to have her back.

Miriam's feeding tube was part of the communication problem. This tube, which was inserted into her mouth and traveled down her throat to her stomach, made it difficult for her to speak and to be understood. The feeding tube also made it difficult to swallow. Since Miriam was no longer receiving hydration intravenously she needed to keep hydrated and water is one of the more difficult things to swallow. One way to maintain hydration was by feeding her applesauce. One of the staff members would try to feed Miriam applesauce a few times an hour. This individual was jokingly known to the family as Mr. Applesauce.

Sara and I also took periodic walks around the hospital and Stanford campus. On one walk that day Sara and I visited the Stanford Art Gallery and museum. My mom had been asking me if I had ever been to the museum. I had not, so here was my chance. We walked all around the museum, which held art and other artifacts, and left. I cannot say that I love museums but I can now say that I have been to the Stanford Museum. After our walk, which was quite pleasant despite the very hot temperature, we returned to the hospital.

The communication difficulties continued. What was occurring, as I understood it, was that Miriam's brain was still recovering from the medications and was foggy. It was very clear that Miriam knew who all of us were and where she was. That was great.

Miriam seemed very tired but she did not want to close her eyes. We tried to talk her into closing her eyes to rest, but she did not cooperate. I can't blame her. If I were in a coma for two weeks I would not want to close my eyes either. Besides her feeding tube she was also hooked up to a few monitors. The machinery was significantly less cumbersome than it was in the ICU. She had access to oxygen if she wanted it which was administered by a mask that she could place over her mouth. We left the hospital after a while to let Miriam rest.

That night before dinner, Sara, Bill and I were having a drink at his home. We had a short while before we were going over to James and Jessica's for dinner. As we were drinking and talking, the topic of Rudy, who is Miriam's brother and only sibling, came up. He had been absent at many of the family's events since he lived a long distance away in New England. I had never met him. When Miriam first entered the hospital a social worker asked her about her family. She mentioned that she had a brother. When the social worker asked her when he would be visiting, Miriam broke down in tears. Her brother would not be visiting, but Bill spoke to Rudy during this trying time on a few occasions. Rudy offered his support and sympathy for his sister.

Bill began to tell stories about Miriam's family.

### The Wedding Party

This story, like all the family stories, takes place in Pennsylvania where Miriam was born and raised. Miriam grew up in the area known as the Lehigh Valley. The Valley's official census area includes Pennsylvania's Lehigh and Northampton Counties and is named for the Lehigh River which runs through it. The Lehigh Valley's principal cities are Allentown, Bethlehem, and Easton, comprising the Allentown-Bethlehem-Easton metropolitan area.

The Lehigh Valley is located approximately 50 miles north of Philadelphia, the country's fifth largest city, and 70 miles west of

New York City, the largest city. The Lehigh Valley is home to some 790,000 people, making it Pennsylvania's third most populated metropolitan region. Recent Pennsylvania census studies show it to be the fastest growing region of Pennsylvania, due mostly to its growing popularity as a bedroom community for the highly-populated neighboring regions of Philadelphia, New Jersey and New York City.

Bill and Miriam were married in California in a small ceremony in picturesque Monterey near the ocean. Because of this, many of Miriam's relatives from Pennsylvania did not attend the wedding. Bill and Miriam planned a reception in Pennsylvania, and they were also celebrating a relative's 85th birthday. Bill and Miriam rented out a restaurant and bar, called Gus's Tavern, and invited a large number of guests.

When the reception and party began there were very few guests and almost all of the guests were women. Hardly any men attended. There was a cake brought to celebrate the event. When the restaurant brought out a cake the servers did not remove the desert from the box. They simply took the box and presented it to the party.

Once the event was over Bill figured out why there were very few guests and why most of these were women. The men and other family members did not attend because they did not want to have to pay to attend the party. The invitation did not specifically state that the party was free for the guests. Bill assumed that the guests would know that they did not have to pay anything to attend the party. On the west coast this point did not need to be written in the invitation. In Pennsylvania it was the custom to make this clear. Life, customs, and assumptions are unique in different parts of the country and world.

**The Funeral**

Another story Bill told involved the funeral for Miriam's mother, Joyce, who tragically passed away from the aftereffects from a car accident. The funeral was to be held in a church that was accessible by a flight of stairs. One of Miriam's aunts, whose name was Pluma, was a rather large woman who could not climb stairs. Miriam asked the pastor of the Lutheran Church if he would hold the service at the funeral home instead of the second floor church. The church did not have adequate facilities to accommodate those with certain physical disabilities or needs. He at first said no. Miriam asked him why. She told the pastor that her children attended Catholic school, and they were always having mass at picnics and other places. The pastor relented and the service was held at the funeral home and Aunt Pluma was able to attend.

A reception following the service was held at the local firehouse. This, like the wedding reception, had a bar which was open and Bill was going to pay the entire tab. Quite a few people were having drinks and enjoying themselves. When Bill went to close out the tab, the total bar bill was a whopping $28. This low price amazed Bill. The cost of living in the Lehigh Valley in Pennsylvania was significantly lower than in the San Francisco Bay Area.

**The Table**

One task that Miriam, Rudy and Bill had after their mother's funeral was to divide up her possessions. One dilemma they had was with, Warren – Miriam's mom's live-in boyfriend. He claimed that he had a life estate to the home, meaning the home was his until he died. Legally the home belonged to Miriam's mother. Warren hired a lawyer who tried to get Bill to communicate with him about the estate. The estate lawyer told Bill that he did not need to communicate with Warren's lawyer. Bill was upset that Warren was taking advantage of the family.

One hot August afternoon in Coopersburg, Pennsylvania, Warren was sitting in a rocking chair in the garage because the home did not have air conditioning. The garage was cooler and provided some relief from the intense heat and stifling humidity. The garage door was open and Bill and Warren were talking.

Warren was trying to give Bill the business card of his lawyer, which he placed on a table. Bill looked at the card and moved his hand towards it as if to pick it up, but instead of picking up the card, he flicked it off the table with his finger. The card fell behind the table. Bill walked out of the garage and borrowed a neighbor's power lawn mower and started to cut the grass. Bill removed the grass catcher from the side of the mower. He cut the patch of grass directly in front of the garage. This created a shower of grass cuttings that covered not only the garage but Warren. Warren jumped out of his rocking chair as angry as could be. Bill kept mowing the lawn, ignoring Warren!

In order to deal with the household items, Bill and Miriam organized an auction. Before the items were going to be available to the general public, they wanted friends and neighbors to get the first chance to purchase anything they might want.

One neighbor, who had been preparing meals for Warren, wanted a particular table and asked the price. Bill said that this person could have the table if she got rid of Warren. Warren vacated the property and dropped his claims to it shortly after this conversation. I am not sure what this neighbor did to get rid of Warren, but Bill was more than happy to give her the table for free. I imagine Warren's lawyer was also asking for payment for his services. This also might have been a factor in dropping the claim.

After these stories we went to James and Jessica's house for dinner. Bill stayed at the hospital that night with Miriam. The hospital brought him a rolling bed and allowed him to stay in the room with her.

# Monday July 4th

*"He who has a why to live can bear almost any how."* -Friedrich Nietzsche

Sara and I left Los Altos and flew to Los Angeles. Before we left we stopped at the hospital to say goodbye to Miriam. We did not have any set plans to return in the near future. We told Miriam that we would call her when we arrived in Los Angeles and we would check in often. Corky took us to the San Jose Airport and a friend, Colleen, picked us up in L.A. and took us to our house. We put away a few things and the three of us walked over to a friend's house to enjoy the Fourth of July holiday. It was chilly, but we still had a pleasant time.

While at our friend's house, Sara called her parents on the phone. It was an absolute miracle that Sara could talk to her mom! A few days earlier Miriam was in a coma and on the brink of death and now they were chatting on the phone. Sara learned that Miriam was eating food that was easy to chew and swallow, plus she was 100% off oxygen. This was more great news. She still had her feeding tube but she was able to chew and swallow soft food.

We enjoyed the fireworks that evening. The City of El Segundo puts on a spectacular fireworks show every Fourth of July.

# Tuesday July 5th

*"Nothing in life is to be feared. It is only to be understood."* -Marie Curie

I spent the greater part of this day trying to get my life back to normal – whatever that was supposed to be. I prepared for the new job I was starting the next day and Sara spent the day getting ready for her tennis classes. I would probably not visit Miriam or our family in Los Altos for at least a few weeks.

We spoke with Bill and he said everything concerning the immediate potential issues were resolved except the feeding tube. Miriam still had it and the doctors were not sure if it was too early to remove. What if she could not properly chew and swallow? What if she was prone to choking? What if there was muscle and tissue damage caused by the coma and the feeding tube? There were a variety of uncertainties concerning the tube. Bill told us that Miriam was going to have a swallowing test later that afternoon, then he was going to report back on the test results.

Later that afternoon we learned that Miriam passed her swallowing test. She could swallow on her own but the doctors were still hesitant to remove the tube. They were going to wait on this decision.

Miriam's memory came and went. She was still extremely confused. She asked my dad how the wedding was over and over again even though there was not a wedding. He answered that the fictitious wedding was splendid. She also asked him what happened to her again and again. He told her what happened each time she asked.

# Wednesday July 6th to Friday July 22nd

*"When you treat a disease, first treat the mind." -Chen Jen*

Sara and I spent the next sixteen days in El Segundo. We received reports about Miriam's condition a few times a day. On July seventh doctors were still not sure what to do about the feeding tube. Perturbed by the indecision, Miriam pulled the tube out herself. Miriam was determined to get it out before the doctors could. She was also determined to get better as soon as she could. She would persevere.

Pulling out the tube was a sign of will, tenacity and the pure desire to heal. I do not think I would have the determination and wherewithal to pull out a tube that could ultimately kill me if my body could not properly move food from the mouth to the stomach. For Miriam, the feeding tube represented something that was holding her back from getting better and exiting the hospital. The removal of the tube did not only have physical significance, but was a symbolic gesture that screamed "I want to get well!" She was healing mentally as well as physically.

A few days later Miriam was moved to the Cancer Center. She'd finally made it back to the place we originally dreaded. This time the Cancer Center was a welcomed and almost celebrated move. She spent a few days at the Cancer Center. During this time she tried to get stronger and was constantly monitored by the team of nurses and doctors. The horrible cancer that almost took her life was still lurking in her system. The blood tests could not locate any cancerous cells and the cancerous mass of tissue had not returned, but the killer was somewhere in her. It was lurking behind healthy cells, waiting for the chance to strike again.

The immediate concern was to improve Miriam's fitness. Her goal was to go home. After spending a few days recuperating in the Cancer Center, Miriam was transferred to the Stanford Hospital Rehabilitation Clinic. Rehab is a place where many of the patients who have been critically injured go before they are released and on their way to recovery. An entire series of books could be dedicated to physical rehab. It is one of the most grueling, intense, frustrating, and rewarding experiences that anyone can experience.

The doctors and nurses design a strict and difficult program tailored for each individual. This could include re-teaching an adult how to talk, how to write their name, how to dress themselves. These sometimes trivial tasks can be some of the most difficult and humiliating actions for someone to do once their body and mind has forgotten how to do them. I will not dwell on rehab any longer but it was a wonderful day and an amazing accomplishment when Miriam completed the tasks put in front of her and was released from the Stanford Hospital Rehabilitation Clinic.

These next few weeks were very sad but also joyous. Miriam was recovering well but the road ahead was uncertain and treacherous. What was certain was that there would be countless challenges. There was discussion about when she would restart chemotherapy, and what drug regiment and combinations would be tried. Would she need surgery to help heal her legs and arms where the blood clots formed? What color and style wig would she like to wear when she loses her hair? We were all delighted, amazed, and grateful that Miriam was out of the ICU and appeared to be on the path to recovery. It had been an incredibly horrible journey so far but the end was not in sight. There was a long way to go but I had witnessed a miracle.

# Saturday July 23rd

*"The human spirit is stronger than anything that can happen to it."*
*-C.C. James*

Miriam went home from the hospital! This was a great day. I was reminded of the deal I made with God on June 23rd, exactly one month prior. On that terrifically horrible day I told God that I would be a better person and live my life in a way that I could help others if he allowed Miriam to survive and make it home, in any way, shape, or form. God held up his end of the deal. Miriam was not only returned to us, she was brought back strong and functioning instead of a helpless invalid. I am working on holding up my end of the deal by being a good person and citizen and trying to help others as much as I can. I know that this is a debt that I will never be able to repay in full, but I am trying.

# The Next Three Years (2005 to 2008)

*"During chemo, you're more tired than you've ever been. It's like a cloud passing over the sun, and suddenly you're out. You don't know how you'll answer the door when your groceries are delivered. But you also find that you're stronger than you've ever been. You're clear. Your mortality is at optimal distance, not up so close that it obscures everything else, but close enough to give you depth perception. Previously, it has taken you weeks, months, or years to discover the meaning of an experience. Now it's instantaneous." -Melissa Bank*

Miriam would spend the greater part of the next three years in and out of Stanford Hospital. There were times where she would need to spend a night or two in the hospital for observation or to receive medication and treatment. Most of the time, however, she received treatment on an outpatient basis. This meant countless trips to the Stanford Cancer Center and hospital. Miriam would receive IVs, blood transfusions, and numerous other medications over the course of her treatment. There would be very good days and there would be awful days.

A PICC line was reinserted in her right arm and remained for most of the treatments. It was extremely important that she kept the PICC line clean and undamaged at all times. Eventually, the PICC line was removed once the intravenous medications were no longer needed. Not having a PICC line was a reason to celebrate.

The major concerns were her reactions to the various treatments, her blood counts and making sure she was not neutropenic. Neutropenia is a blood disorder where the white blood cell count is low. When this occurs the patient is especially susceptible to infections. These infections are life threatening. When Miriam was neutropenic she had to wear her mask, stay away from people as much as possible, and only eat food prepared in the home. This was to ensure that she knew exactly what she was eating and that the food was cooked well done. It was imperative that as many germs, viruses and other food-borne occurrences were killed before they were consumed.

In preparation for Miriam's return home, Bill installed handrails at the entry ways to make it easier and safer for Miriam to navigate. Bill called his friend John to inquire who installed stainless steel ADA handrails in John's home when his wife was in a similar state from cancer prior to her passing away from the disease. At 9:30am John returned Bill's call. He told Bill that he would give him the handrails. Bill met John and one of John's employees at 10:30 at his home. The employee took out the railings at John's home and installed them at Bill's. This is what it means to be a friend. He completed the job by 1:00 that afternoon.

The handrails made it easier and safer for Miriam to enter and exit their home. These were helpful since she was frail and susceptible to falling. The drugs and treatments have worn down her bones and made her muscles ache. This is a lasting effect of cancer treatment that is still prevalent today.

Also, because of the complication of the blood clot that formed in Miriam's leg, she required surgery to graft skin on the wound. Miriam went back into the hospital for a week to complete this procedure. This was extremely risky but necessary. Because of her low white blood count the wound did not heal quickly and the fear of infection was high. Miriam still has a scar on her leg from the blood clot and surgery.

During her rehabilitation for the skin graft, Bill ran into Doctor Montoya, chief of the infectious disease division at Stanford. Doctor Montoya was personally in charge of Miriam while she was in the intensive care unit. He also provided her with medication and drugs to help reduce the chance of infection or disease while she was neutropenic. Doctor Montoya was a wonderful resource during treatment. Bill told Doctor Montoya that Stanford Hospital produced a miracle in saving Miriam's life. Doctor Montoya responded matter-of-factly, "Yes, we did play a role. Your wife had a 5% chance of survival. The first night in the ICU we almost lost her three times. As far as miracles go, there was a higher calling that saved Miriam."

# 2008 – 2012

*"The future is literally in our hands to mold as we like. But we cannot wait until tomorrow. Tomorrow is now." -Eleanor Roosevelt*

As the seconds, minutes, hours, days, weeks, months and years passed, Sara and I were updated on Miriam's conditions, trials and tribulations. We visited as often as we could and always tried to keep informed of the latest information and developments. Miriam took each milestone, setback, and turn in the road with a positive attitude and an unfathomable strength. She is a warrior in all senses of the word.

Miriam's hair has grown back, her strength has returned, she is back on the tennis court, and she has finished all cancer treatments. Hopefully the horrible cancer that came extremely close to taking her life multiple times will not return. If it does, I know Miriam will be ready to fight like hell again, and again, and again.

As of 2012 Miriam is officially cancer free and has celebrated her 65th birthday. The cancer cannot be found and she does not need to visit specialists or spend time at the hospital. She has five grandchildren and a social schedule that keeps her busy. Sara's sister Jessica has four children, and my wife and I have one. Jessica's oldest, Sammy, is eight. The word cancer is brought up less and less often in our family, yet I know it is always on our minds. Cancer is a horrible disease. Miriam is extremely lucky to have been able to beat this monster. This would not have been possible without the unbending support of doctors, nurses, friends, family and God. The debt we owe Stanford Hospital and its staff can never be repaid. Hopefully this book will help those who are affected by cancer's grip. There is always hope.

*"Don't give up. Don't ever give up." -Jim Valvano*

## Acknowledgements

I would like to extend a special thank you to my family and friends and especially Marilyn, Ron, Maureen, Al, Matt, Katy, Shane and Father Gary. Also, thank you to Sean Hooks for your editorial expertise and Rene Quebec for your design excellence. This is dedicated to everyone who has been touched by cancer. Unfortunately, this is a very large number.

## Select Sources

Thank you to the internet. Without you, this would have been a more difficult endeavor to complete.

- http://www.cancernet.co.uk/poems.htm
- http://www.cancer.org/Research/CancerFactsFigures/index
- http://www.cancer.org/acs/groups/content/ @epidemiologysurveilance/documents/document/ acspc-032674.pptx
- http://www.cancer.org/acs/groups/content/ @epidemiologysurveilance/documents/document/ acspc-031941.pdf
- http://www.mayoclinic.com/health/chemotherapy/ MY00536
- http://www.tvland.com/shows/mash/episode-guide/ season-8
- http://stanfordhospital.org/

- http://stanfordhospital.org/newsEvents/newsReleases/2011/us-news-world-report.html
- http://stanfordhospital.org/aboutUs/facts.html
- http://www.usacitiesonline.com/cacountyelsegundo.htm
- http://en.wikipedia.org/wiki/Los_Altos,_California
- http://en.wikipedia.org/wiki/Neutrophil_granulocyte
- http://en.wikipedia.org/wiki/T-cell_leukemia
- http://en.wikipedia.org/wiki/Peripherally_inserted_central_catheter
- http://en.wikipedia.org/wiki/Hemostasis
- http://www.relayforlife.org/

## About the Author

Jordan Lane lives with his wife and daughter in El Segundo, California. He is also the author of *The Babysitting Bible*. Jordan holds a bachelor's degree in History and a master's degree in Public Administration. Find Jordan online at *www.52daysTheCancerJournal.com* and on Twitter @JordanDLane.